Get Through

MRCGP: AKT

Library (MEC), Queens Hospital Burton
library.bur@burtonh-tr.wmids.nhs.uk

Contents

Preface

The new MRCGP (nMRCGP) applied knowledge test (AKT) is a multiple choice question exam of 200 items carried out over 3 hours. It is an exam which, I believe, every candidate is capable of passing. The question is, how do you make sure you go into the exam knowing you have prepared to the best of your ability?

In this book, I have concentrated on the themes and subjects which candidates often answer poorly. It is improvement in a candidate's areas of weakness that will allow them to pass the exam. To this end I have included extended explanations in the answers section, especially in subjects where candidates often perform poorly. The reason for this is to allow candidates to gain confidence answering these more challenging questions, which may be the crucial ones in any exam. A book containing only very easy questions, while encouraging to morale to some extent, probably would not be much actual use as a revision tool! Therefore, as the content of these questions is focussed towards these more challenging areas, don't expect perfection when doing these questions, at least initially!

I have split the questions into papers of 100, rather than the 200 questions you will face in the exam. This is merely for practical reasons, to have groups of questions in manageable chunks. I have not set a pass mark because I feel this would be rather arbitrary; however, if you are getting marks above 60%, or nearing the approximation of 70% required to pass the real exam, you are well on your way to success.

I have not included photo questions here for two reasons: (1) Printing photos would have made the book prohibitively expensive; (2) Your photographic identification skills should come from your own clinical experience. If you would prefer to spend some time revising signs you are not likely to have come across in clinical practice, an atlas of clinical signs from your practice library should help in this regard.

I hope you find this book useful. It has been compiled immediately following my own nMRCGP experience, and includes some of the information gathered during my own revision, which I found was not readily available in a single textbook. While I can't claim this as a complete and comprehensive guide to all potential subjects in the AKT, I have tried to make it representative of the material that is most relevant to anyone embroiled in the stressful task of working out both what to study and how to study for the AKT.

All the best!

Dianne Campbell

AKT strategies

The secret to passing this exam is to work *smart*, not just *hard*. There are thousands of multiple choice questions available from various sources for the exam candidate. Because of this, a possible pitfall would be to do hundreds of questions, continually congratulating yourself on the ones you got right, but doing nothing about the ones you get wrong. This strategy is, of course, little benefit in increasing your potential exam score.

My recommendation would be to make a note of things you are unsure of or questions you want to go back to, as you go through sets of practice questions such as in this book. It is better to spend time improving your understanding of one question, than to look at 20 questions to which you already know the answers.

Also, as you revise, you will become aware of facts and topics you will want to go over just before the exam. I found it useful to put some of these 'last minute facts' on index cards to use as flash cards before the exam. The strength of these is that their size means you can't waste time making extensive notes, and they can be flipped through very quickly. Everyone's list will be different, but here are some subjects you may find useful to go over just before the exam:

- Definitions of sensitivity, specificity, negative and positive predictive values
- Blood pressure targets
- Details of Med3, Med4 certificates, etc.
- COPD treatment steps
- Asthma treatment steps
- DVLA guidelines
- Benefit details – jobseekers, disability living allowance, etc.
- Child development milestones.

As well as doing lots of practice questions, I would recommend speed reading the first 100 or so pages of the *Oxford Handbook of General Practice*, bearing in mind that this is one of the core curriculum texts as designated by the RCGP. It has all of the information required to handle the management questions in the exam. Candidates often do poorly in these questions because of a relative lack of exposure to management issues in training.

Finally, try to think of as many potential algorithm questions as possible. These are generally treatment algorithms, so look at local and national guidelines to try to second guess what might be used in the exam. Topics which lend themselves to algorithm questions include:

- COPD treatments steps
- Asthma treatment steps
- Fertility investigation pathway
- GI bleeding patient pathway
- Dyspepsia patient pathway
- Obesity treatment pathway
- Irregular menstrual bleeding patient pathway

- Breast lump treatment algorithm
- Prostate assessment algorithm
- Pain management pathway
- Menorrhagia algorithm
- Addictions treatment algorithms.

Also remember that the details of some of the legislation that forms part of the curriculum for the AKT may vary slightly between the four countries that make up the UK (i.e. Scotland, Northern Ireland, Wales and England). Broadly speaking, the principles surrounding the Mental Capacity Acts and the Mental Health Acts are the same but the section numbers pertaining to each subject differ. The Royal College of General Practitioners' official statement on the subject suggests that as a licensing exam for GPs to work all around the country, candidates should be familiar with legislation from all countries. It would seem unlikely, however, that an AKT question about the Mental Health Act (Scotland) would come up in a UK-wide AKT paper. It is much more likely that in areas of the curriculum where there are differences between countries, questions would be constructed to assess legislation that is the same in all parts of the UK. In time, the AKT may be constructed to differ depending where in the country you are sitting the exam, but there is no suggestion of this at present.

Practical points

Be on time. This is an exam with extremely strict rules. If you forget your passport or other prescribed identification **you will not be allowed in**. Read your instructions carefully as they are strictly enforced.

The exam is carried out on computer and consists of questions from 1 to 200. There is the opportunity to 'flag' a particular question by ticking a box, which allows you to come back directly to that question. If you choose to do this, it is highly advisable to put a tick in one of the boxes as a 'guess answer'. Time is tight in this exam and it is possible that you will not have sufficient time to go back over every question. However, if you do have enough time you can return to any question, not only those you have 'flagged'.

No food or water is allowed in the exam. No electronic devices including watches are allowed.

You will be supplied with a double-sided, laminated sheet of paper and a non-permanent pen. This is useful for carrying out quick calculations.

Unless otherwise stated, the questions are asking for a 'best of five' answer, i.e. selecting one correct response from five possible ones. If you are required to give more than one answer, it will be clear. The computer will only allow you to enter the required number of answers and no more.

Finally, remember that although you may, in preparing for this exam, worry excessively about the minutiae, this is ultimately an exam testing a candidate's competence to practise. While this book is an aid to preparing for the exam, like all academic pursuits, it is secondary to solid practical experience in medical practice.

Acknowledgements

I would like to thank the following for their contributions to this book and for time spent proof reading and fact checking:

Mrs Ashlyne Buchan – Advanced Practitioner Radiographer, St Mary's Hospital, Isle of Wight

Dr Ashok Jacob – Consultant Cardiologist, St John's Hospital, Livingston

Dr Anshuman Sengupta – Foundation doctor, Edinburgh

Dr Adrian Palfreeman – Consultant in GU Medicine, Leicester Royal Infirmary

Dr Roddy Campbell – Consultant Pathologist, Monklands Hospital, Coatbridge

Dr Amanda Fairman – GP, Edinburgh

Dr Anne Aulmann – GP, Edinburgh

Dr David Atkinson – GP, Edinburgh

Dr David Smith – GP, Edinburgh

Dr Panagiotis Roupakiotis – GP, Edinburgh

Dr D J MacInnes – GP, Edinburgh

Dr Fiona Easton – GP, Edinburgh

Gareth Evans – Royal Navy GP

Dr Jill Ferguson – GP, Edinburgh

Dr Joanna Loudon – GP, Edinburgh

Dr Katherine McInroy – GP, West Lothian

Dr Laura Serafini – GP, Edinburgh

Dr Leona Carroll – GP, Edinburgh

Dr Lorna Goldring – GP, Edinburgh

Dr Maria Simon-Marin – GP, Edinburgh

Dr Sarah Little – GP, West Lothian

Dr Keith Russell – GP Principal, West Lothian

Dr Greig Carlaw – GP Principal, West Lothian

Dr Jackie Lees – GP Principal, West Lothian

Dr James McCallum – GP Principal, West Lothian

Dr Fergus McRae – GP Principal, West Lothian

Dr David Molyneux – Fellow in Medical Ethics, Department of Postgraduate Medicine and Dentistry, University of Manchester

Dr Helen Turner – GP, West Lothian

Thanks to the Sarahs Burrows and Vasey and the editing publishing team at RSM, and also the team at Naughton Project Management, for their patience and help. Thanks to all at Newland Medical Practice in Bathgate, the best training Practice in the country in my own humble opinion.

Thanks also to my family, friends, including the King's Church Motherwell and Monklands for their unwavering support and babysitting. I am blessed to have you all.

For my wonderful husband Roddy
and my beautiful son Daniel:
my greatest gifts

1) *Red flag signs*

A 45-year-old woman on your list presents to you for the first time in 5 years. She has a 2-week history of new symptoms.

Which ONE of the following is LEAST likely to be associated with a sinister diagnosis?

A Haematuria
B Haemoptysis
C Dysphagia
D Menorrhagia
E Rectal bleeding

2) *Treatment of angina*

One of your patients attends A&E with a first episode of cardiac chest pain. Subsequent exercise tolerance testing confirms stable angina.

Which ONE of the following is the first line treatment for symptomatic relief AND mortality reduction?

A GTN spray
B Calcium channel blocker
C Beta-blocker
D ACE inhibitor
E Long-acting nitrates

3–10) *Treatment of psoriasis*

A 23-year-old woman with severe chronic plaque psoriasis has attended your surgery to discuss possible treatments before considering referral to a dermatologist.

Match the following list of drugs with the statements below.

A Acitretin
B Betamethasone 0.1%
C Calcipotriol
D Coal tar
E Ciclosporin
F Dithranol
G Hydrocortisone 2.5%
H Methotrexate
I UVB
J UVA
K Tazarotene

3) Messy, topical treatment that can irritate the skin. Contains known carcinogens.

4) Systemic treatment for severe psoriasis unresponsive to conventional therapy. Uses weekly dosing.

5) Systemic treatment where pregnancy should be avoided for at least 2 years after stopping therapy due to teratogenic risk.

6) Systemic treatment for severe psoriasis unresponsive to conventional therapy. Uses daily dosing. Side effects include gum hypertrophy, hypertension and kidney damage.

7) Messy, topical treatment that can irritate the skin. Usually applied for a 'short contact' and washed off after 5–60 minutes. Causes permanent staining of bedding and clothes. Not suitable for use on flexures.

8) A topical vitamin D analogue.

9) Used with psoralens to treat psoriasis.

10) Potent topical steroid used when less potent steroids have been ineffective.

11–16) *Ethical principles*
In the following scenarios identify the MOST important ethical principle involved:

A Autonomy
B Beneficence
C Non-maleficence
D Informed consent
E Confidentiality
F Justice

11) A 32-year-old woman with known asthma attends the out-of-hours service. She is presenting for the fifth time this year due to a panic attack with palpitations. Her chest is clear on examination with no respiratory distress. The doctor on duty suggests using propranolol to help deal with her panic attacks.

12) A 15-year-old girl wants a definite guarantee that her parents will not find out that she wants to go onto the contraceptive injection.

13) A 35-year-old woman campaigns to have her local health authority fund a new treatment for breast cancer, which has evidence of benefit, but is very expensive. This treatment is available in her neighbouring city.

14) A patient feels pressured into attending for a smear test.

15) A 60-year-old man collapses in the waiting room. Resuscitation is commenced and an ambulance called.

16) A 70-year-old lady in a nursing home has been told by her family that her doctor has given her a sleeping tablet. The tablet the lady is taking at night is in fact her simvastatin. The belief in her sleeping tablet has improved her sleep pattern.

17) *Ethical theory*
On which of the following is our framework of autonomy, beneficence, non-maleficence, confidentiality and informed consent based?

A Ethical relativism
B Divine command theory
C Utilitarianism
D Deontology
E Virtue ethics

18) *Specificity and sensitivity*
The specificity of a test is:

A The number of true negatives detected by the test divided by the true positives in the population tested

B The proportion of true positives detected by the test divided by the true positives in the population tested

C The proportion of true negatives detected by the test divided by the true negatives in the population tested

D The number of true negatives detected by the test divided by the true negatives in the population tested

E The number of true positives detected by the test divided by the true positives in the population tested

19) *Crossover trials*
Which of the following is true regarding a crossover trial?

A It is useful for comparing treatments for acute urinary tract infection

B It cannot be adequately randomized

C It cannot be adequately blinded

D It tends to need more subjects than with other trial designs to achieve adequate power

E It is useful for comparing analgesia treatment for chronic osteoarthritis

20–24) *Peripheral neuropathies*
For each of the following clinical scenarios, select the most likely diagnosis. Each option may be used once, more than once or not at all:

A Charcot–Marie–Tooth disease

B Cisplatin therapy

C Diabetic neuropathy

D Guillain–Barré syndrome

E Multiple compression palsy

F Multiple sclerosis

G Systematic vasculitis

20) A 30-year-old man presents with distal paraesthesia and distal weakness occurring 1–2 weeks after a GI infection. The reflexes are present initially but become absent within 1 hour. He soon loses the ability to walk and develops facial and bulbar weakness.

21) A 70-year-old woman with rheumatoid arthritis presents with rapid onset of multiple mononeuropathy.

22) A 30-year-old male patient with a history of metastatic seminoma presents with months of ataxia. He has been undergoing chemotherapy. He states that his gait is worse in the dark. No other member of his family has a history of similar symptoms. He has also noticed occasional arm weakness. He has no history of back pain and a recent bone scan showed no evidence of bone metastasis. Examination shows a lower motor neurone lesion.

23) A 15-year-old male presents with a bilateral weakness in his lower limbs. On examination he has foot drop, pes cavus and claw toes. His mother had the same symptoms in her twenties.

24) A 60-year-old obese man who rarely attends his surgery presents with a painful peripheral neuropathy with a stocking and glove distribution. On examination he has a poorly healing ulcer on the ball of his left foot.

25–28) *Study design*

Match the following studies with the most appropriate study design for the following study questions:

A Case-control study
B Cohort study
C Cross-sectional study
D Meta-analysis (Forest plot)
E Randomized controlled study

25) A study following up the eventual career choices of groups of first year medical students from universities in England and Scotland.

26) A study to determine the percentage of babies born to mothers treated with thalidomide who developed limb hypoplasia.

27) A survey of five GP practices' antiviral prescribing habits.

28) A comparison of trials looking at the risk of DVT with third-generation combined oral contraceptives.

29) *Notification of death*
Which of the following deaths DO NOT need to be reported to the coroner?

A Death through neglect
B Death due to industrial disease
C Death due to chronic alcoholism
D Deceased not attended by a doctor in their last illness
E Death due to suspected suicide

30) *Treatment of acute psychosis*
You see a 40-year-old mature student at home at the request of his wife because he has been having auditory hallucinations. His acute psychosis is managed in hospital where he is diagnosed with acute schizophrenia.
Upon discharge, he should be maintained on:

A Clozapine
B Haloperidol
C Olanzapine
D Piportil
E Pimozide

31–35) *ECG changes*
Match the following descriptions of ECG abnormalities with the correct diagnosis:

A Acute myocardial infarction
B Low potassium level
C High calcium level
D Acute pericarditis
E Pulmonary embolus

31) Q waves in leads II, III, aVF with ST elevation and T wave inversion.

32) Deep S waves in lead I, pathological Q waves in lead III and inverted T wave in lead III.

33) Concave, saddle-shaped, ST segment elevation.

34) Prolonged QT interval.

35) Shortened QT interval.

36) *Otitis media*

You see an 18-month-old baby in the GP out-of-hours service. She presents with a 36-hour history of right earache and high fever. On examination, her temperature is 39°C and the tympanic membrane is red and bulging.

The most appropriate treatment is:

A Amoxicillin
B Ibuprofen
C Paracetamol
D Reassurance and review
E Gentisone ear drops

37) *Notifiable diseases*

A 38-year-old man presents with diarrhoea and vomiting 1 week after returning from travel to Africa. He did not take malaria pro-phylaxis and has had a Chinese takeaway meal 3 days ago, which he thinks may have given him food poisoning. You undertake to identify possible infections causing this man's illness.

Which of the following diseases DOES NOT have to be reported to Public Health?

A Dysentery
B Salmonellosis
C Viral gastroenteritis
D Haemorrhagic fever
E Malaria

38) *Industrial injury*

A 23-year-old nurse attends your surgery having hurt her back at work. She tried to lift a patient on her own and immediately felt her 'back go'. She has been off work due to this injury for 1 week and has attended because she would like you to issue a Med3 certificate. She feels she is not adequately supported at work. **Which of the following types of injury DOES NOT need to be reported by the employer to the Health and Safety Executive?**

A Dangerous incidents, even if no one was injured
B Injury where death occurred
C Incidents where injury causes 2 days absence from work
D Incidents involving gas
E Injury where the employee did not follow safety procedures

39) *Nicotine replacement therapy*
A 19-year-old woman attends your surgery asking about nicotine replacement therapy. She has an extensive past medical history including psoriasis and diabetes. Two months later, she attends your surgery because she has just found out she is pregnant. She wants to discuss her continued use of nicotine replacement therapy. **Contraindications to nicotine replacement therapy include all of the following EXCEPT:**

A Breastfeeding
B Chronic psoriasis
C Diabetes mellitus
D Previously failed smoking attempt
E Ongoing cigarette smoking

40) *Alopecia*
The following conditions may be associated with alopecia EXCEPT:

A Chronic iron deficiency
B Fungal scalp infection
C Hyperthyroidism
D Polycystic ovarian syndrome
E Warfarin

41) *Diabetic retinopathy*
Which of the following is most likely to be present in diabetic retinopathy?

A Flame retinal haemorrhage
B Grey opalescent retina
C Arteriovenous nipping
D Microaneurysms
E Optic neuritis

42) *Hypertensive retinopathy*
Which of the following is most likely to be seen in hypertensive retinopathy?

A Yellow hard exudates
B Grey opalescent retina
C Arteriovenous nipping
D Microaneurysms
E Optic neuritis

43–45) *Management of mental illness*
For each of the following patients, select the most appropriate course of action:

A Continue antidepressant for 2 more weeks
B Increase the dose of antidepressant or consider switching to another
C Prescribe antipsychotic
D Prescribe antidepressant
E Refer to psychiatric outpatient clinic
F Urgent referral for admission

43) The mother of a 20-year-old unemployed man is concerned, since her son has not left his room for 3 months. The son agrees for you to visit him at home and during your visit you find him aloof. You determine that he does not have psychotic features.

44) You are contacted by the neighbour of a 25-year-old woman. You contact the woman, who agrees for you to visit her at home. Upon arrival you see that there is broken window glass, used syringes and beer bottles scattered on the floor. She reports that she cannot sleep as she hears shouting voices in her head.

45) A 35-year-old man on Prozac states that nothing has happened in 6 weeks. He asks whether he can try a different antidepressant.

46) *Drugs requiring monitoring*
A new patient attends your surgery for a new patient medical. He has chronic obstructive pulmonary disease (COPD), a history of cardiovascular disease and gout. He cannot remember which drugs he is on but he knows he has to have regular blood tests to check the level in his blood.
Which of the following requires regular blood drug level testing?

A Warfarin
B Atenolol
C Theophylline
D Bendroflumethiazide
E Tiotropium

47–54) *Consultation models*

Match the following authors with their described consultation models:

A Byrne and Long
B Stott and Davis
C Pendleton et al.
D Neighbour
E Calgary–Cambridge observation guide
F Tuckett et al.
G Helman
H Balint
I Berne

47) Patients' health beliefs

48) The doctor, his patient and the illness: the doctor as a drug.

49) The inner consultation: five signposts in a consultation

50) The exceptional potential in each primary care consultation

51) Transactional analysis – games people play. Parent, adult and child ego states

52) The consultation: seven tasks

53) The meeting of two experts

54) Doctors talking to patients: six logical steps to a consultation

55) *GMS contract*

You are deciding which services are appropriate to provide within your practice. Which of the following is an essential service within the GP GMS contract?

A Cervical screening
B Child health surveillance
C Maternity services
D Contraceptive services
E Terminal illness

56) *Consultation rates*
Which of the following factors are known to INCREASE consultation rates in general practice?

A Personal lists within a practice
B Social deprivation
C High practice list size
D School summer holidays
E Not prescribing antibiotics for otitis media

57) *Data Protection Act 1998*
A patient of yours wishes to see their medical records. Which of the following does the patient have the right to see?

A Information more than 2 years old
B Information in her record which refers to a third person
C Information which may cause mental or physical harm
D Information where the patient cannot be directly identified
E The medical record of her deceased husband as she suspects he had an affair prior to his death. She was his next of kin

58) *Removal from practice list*
You attend a practice meeting. The first item on the agenda is to discuss whether a particular patient should be removed from the practice list.
Which of the following is NOT an appropriate reason for removal from a practice list?

A Violence
B Deliberately lying about a home address
C A patient moves to a new address outwith the practice area.
D Repeated refusal of a patient to accept a GP's advice
E Removal of another household member from the practice list

59) *Ionising Radiation (Medical Exposure) Regulations*
Regarding X-ray referrals, which of the following is NOT part of the Ionising Radiation (Medical Exposure) Regulations?

A A non-ionizing radiation method of imaging should be used wherever possible
B The examination should be justified on the basis of the clinical information provided
C Adequate clinical information should be included to make this decision
D The benefits should outweigh the radiation risks
E Responsibility for minimizing radiation exposure lies solely with the referrer

60) *Cervical spine X-ray*
You are sending a 50-year-old patient for a cervical spine X-ray.
Which of the following indications is most appropriate?

A Dizziness
B Acute torticollis
C Cervical rib
D Atlanto-axial subluxation in a patient with rheumatoid arthritis prior to a general anaesthetic
E Degenerative change

61) *Faith considerations*
Below is a list of considerations which may apply regarding health-care. To which one of the following World Faiths might these apply?

- Many followers will be vegetarian. Medications should be offered suitable for vegetarians.
- A new mother will rest for 40 days after the birth of a new baby. Female relatives may want to care for the child while in hospital to help the mother rest.
- A priest may be called upon to select an appropriate name for the child. This will be given to the child at a naming ceremony. Both the temporary birth name and the planned name should be recorded in the child's clinical records.
- When a patient dies, the family is likely to want to return the body of their dead relative to the earth as quickly as possible, usually by cremation. The ashes will be scattered at a later date into a river (preferably the River Ganges in India).

A Buddhism
B Hinduism
C Islam
D Judaism
E Sikhism

62) *Nystagmus*
A 35-year-old patient attends your surgery complaining of dizziness. This has come on over the past 24 hours following a cold 1 week ago. She has vomited. On examination, she has horizontal nystagmus which is more pronounced when looking to the left. The nystagmus disappears when she looks straight ahead.
Where are her symptoms likely to be coming from?

A Brain stem
B Right middle ear
C Right cerebellum
D Left middle ear
E Left cerebellum

63) *Benzodiazepines*

A 45-year-old woman attends your surgery. She started taking temazepam at night following the death of her husband 5 years ago, and she has never been able to stop. She is now keen to come off and would like to be gradually cut down. She takes 20 mg temazepam at bedtime. To start the withdrawal, her dose is converted to diazepam.

How much diazepam is equivalent to 20 mg temazepam at night?

A 5 mg diazepam
B 10 mg diazepam
C 20 mg diazepam
D 40 mg diazepam
E 80 mg diazepam

64) *Morphine prescribing*

A 61-year-old man is suffering from oesophageal carcinoma. He is finding he is unable to swallow his morphine analgesia.

When switching to subcutaneous infusion of morphine, what dose is used compared to the 24-hour oral dose?

A $\frac{1}{4}$ total 24-hour oral morphine dose

B $\frac{1}{3}$ total 24-hour oral morphine dose

C $\frac{1}{2}$ total 24-hour oral morphine dose

D $\frac{2}{3}$ total 24-hour oral morphine dose

E Equal to total 24-hour oral morphine dose

65) *Disease-modifying agents in rheumatoid arthritis*

A 50-year-old woman has longstanding rheumatoid arthritis. She has been on a number of drugs for this and has had to stop treatment with both sulfasalazine and methotrexate. She has been on indometacin for the past 3 years but is now finding that it is upsetting her stomach.

What is the SINGLE next best treatment to try?

A Ciclosporin
B Leflunomide
C Misoprostol
D Naproxen
E Celecoxib

66–71) *Asthma diagnosis in adults*

Complete the following algorithm regarding the diagnosis of asthma in adults by selecting an answer from the list below for each numbered box.

A Further investigation. Consider referral
B Continue treatment
C FEV1/FVC < 0.7
D Assess compliance and inhaler technique. Consider further investigation and/or referral
E FEV1/FVC > 0.7

Diagnosis of asthma is a clinical one based on a characteristic symptom pattern and lack of an alternative diagnosis

Investigation of adults presenting with suspected asthma. (Reproduced by kind permission of The British Thoracic Society and Scottish Intercollegiate Guidelines Network. British Guideline on the Management of Asthma. May 2008.)

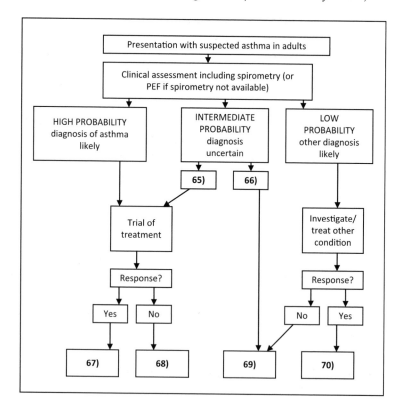

72–77) *Forest plot interpretation*

The Forest plot below shows a meta-analysis of trials testing a new drug to improve airflow in COPD.

A Study A
B Study B
C Study C
D Study D
E Study E
F 1
G 2
H 3
I 4
J 5
K Meta-analysis shows overall benefit
L Meta-analysis shows overall harm
M Meta-analysis shows overall no difference

Forest plot

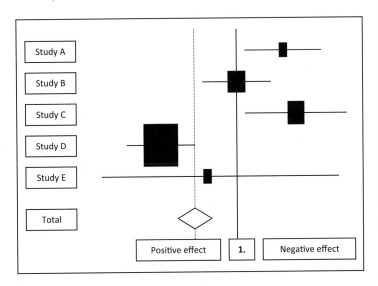

72) Which study most strongly shows evidence of benefit of the drug in treating COPD?

73) Which study most strongly shows evidence of harm of the drug in treating COPD?

74) Which study has the highest power in the meta-analysis?

75) Which study has the widest confidence intervals?

76) How many studies show a statistically significant benefit?

77) What is the overall outcome of the meta-analysis?

78) *Doctor's bag*
When carrying a doctor's bag containing drugs during home visits, which is considered by the police to be the lowest acceptable level of security?

A Storing an unlocked bag in a locked car
B Storing a lockable bag in the boot of a locked car
C Storing a locked bag in the back seat of a locked car
D Storing a locked bag in the boot of a locked car
E Storing an unlocked bag in the back of an unlocked car

79) *Thyroid cancers*
Which single type of malignant thyroid cancer is the most common?

A Anaplastic
B Follicular
C Medullary
D Lymphoma
E Papillary

80) *Dementia*
A 75-year-old man has a 3-month history of general deterioration in his ability to look after himself, with recurrent falls. He has also had episodes of confusion, claiming not to recognize his wife. He has called the police on more than one occasion because he believes his house is under attack from giant insects. His only medication is bendrofluazide and aspirin. On examination, he has an expressionless face but no cranial nerve lesions. His gait is slow and shuffling. He has increased tone in all limbs.
What is the most likely diagnosis?

A Parkinson's disease
B Progressive supranuclear palsy
C Multi-system atrophy
D Lewy body dementia
E Schizophrenia

81) *Factitious seizures*

A 19-year-old woman has had recurrent seizures, which have been resistant to treatment. You suspect factitious seizures.

Which one of the following is most likely to suggest this?

A The ability to be talked or calmed out of a seizure
B Seizure only when no one is present
C Duration of less than 2 minutes
D Preserved consciousness during a seizure
E Speech during a seizure

82) *Causes of seizure*

You see an 80-year-old woman with her son in your emergency surgery following a short seizure that day. This is her first seizure. Her son reports that she has become increasingly confused over the past 2 weeks. She is now struggling to look after herself and he has been coming over to make her meals. On examination, she is a little drowsy with no fever and a BP 195/111. She has a mild hemiparesis on examination. Her son is not aware of her having fallen recently.

What is the most likely diagnosis?

A Meningitis
B Transient ischaemic attack
C Cerebrovascular accident
D Acute intracerebral haemorrhage
E Subdural haematoma

83) *Liver enzyme-inducing drugs*

A 23-year-old woman is considering taking the oral contraceptive pill (OCP). She is on a number of different medications already.

Which of the following drugs may cause the OCP to fail due to liver enzyme induction?

A Omeprazole
B Valproate
C Carbamazepine
D Cimetidine
E Evening primrose oil

84) *Liver enzyme inhibition*
A 65-year-old woman has been on warfarin for 5 years. At her routine INR check, her INR has nearly doubled. Her warfarin is immediately stopped.
Looking back at her medical record, commencement of which of the following drugs would be most likely to raise her INR due to liver enzyme inhibition?

A Erythromycin
B Rifampicin
C Oxytetracycline
D Trimethoprim
E Cefalexin

85) *Medication side effects*
A 70-year-old woman presents with swollen lower legs. She is on 5 mg felodipine for hypertension and indometacin for rheumatic disease. Her BP is currently 140/70.
The SINGLE most appropriate step is:

A Add a loop diuretic
B Add a thiazide diuretic
C Change felodipine to an ACE inhibitor
D Change indometacin to a COX-2 inhibitor
E Prescribe elastic stockings

86–91) *Diabetes diagnosis*
For each of the following test situations, match the appropriate answer for a positive test result:

A One test ≥ 6.1 mmol/l
B Two tests ≥ 6.1 mmol/l
C One test ≥ 7.0 mmol/l
D Two tests ≥ 7.0 mmol/l
E One test ≥ 7.8 mmol/l
F Two tests ≥ 7.8 mmol/l
G One test ≥ 11.1 mmol/l
H Two tests ≥ 11.1 mmol/l

86) To diagnose diabetes using an oral glucose tolerance test following fasting glucose.

87) To diagnose diabetes using a fasting blood glucose if symptomatic.

88) To diagnose diabetes using a fasting blood glucose if asymptomatic.

89) To diagnose diabetes using random blood glucose measurements if symptomatic.

90) To diagnose diabetes using random blood glucose measurements if asymptomatic.

91) To diagnose impaired glucose tolerance test using an oral glucose tolerance test following fasting glucose.

92–98) *Obesity*

Match the following scenarios regarding obesity guidelines with their matching body mass index:

A BMI > 26
B BMI > 27
C BMI > 28
D BMI > 30
E BMI > 35
F BMI > 40
G BMI > 50

92) Prescribe orlistat only in adults if

93) Prescribe orlistat only in adults with diabetes and

94) Prescribe sibutramine or rimonabant only in adults if

95) Prescribe sibutramine or rimonabant only in adults with diabetes and

96) Patients can be referred for bariatric surgery following drug therapy if

97) Patients can be referred for bariatric surgery following drug therapy if they are hypertensive and

98) Patients can be referred for bariatric surgery first line if

99) *Menopause*

A 50-year-old woman reports night sweats and hot flushes. **Which blood test would you order to confirm menopause?**

A FSH
B LH
C Progesterone
D Prolactin
E Testosterone

100) *Amenorrhoea*

A 19-year-old female patient presents with amenorrhoea of 6 months' duration. She is currently a law student in her second year. Since starting university she has joined the union running club and is training for the local marathon. She is currently running 9 miles daily. She feels she has been under a lot of stress but does not feel depressed. Her menarche was at 14 and she had regular periods till 2 years ago when they became irregular. Her BMI is 20 and she has not lost any weight recently.

The most likely cause of her amenorrhoea is:

A Pregnancy
B Over-exercising
C Premature ovarian failure
D Polycystic ovarian syndrome
E Stress

1) D Menorrhagia

This question is frustrating because you want to know more about the patient's symptoms. The question is testing your knowledge of classic red flag signs so use the bare facts you are given. Haemoptysis and rectal bleeding are the most obvious red flag signs. Dysphagia with weight loss and painless frank haematuria are also red flag signs. Postmenopausal bleeding is a red flag sign but menorrhagia on its own is very unlikely to be sinister.

2) C Beta-blocker

A beta-blocker is first line treatment for both symptoms and reducing mortality. Neither calcium channel blockers nor nitrates have any evidence for reducing mortality, but they both help symptoms. If beta-blockers cannot be tolerated, use a calcium channel blocker to help symptoms. ACE inhibitors are used to reduce overall cardiovascular risk, which should be a priority in treating this patient.

When considering reduction of cardiovascular risk consider:
- lifestyle, especially smoking
- blood pressure
- blood glucose
- aspirin
- statin.

3) D Coal tar

Coal tar contains polycyclic aromatic hydrocarbon – known carcinogens. Tolerated poorly by outpatients because of the mess involved. Can be irritating, especially if inflammation present.

4) H Methotrexate

Methotrexate should be prescribed with folic acid to reduce the risk of toxicity. Advice to reduce the risk of drug error is to dispense one strength tablets only. The patient is warned to report any signs of possible toxicity, e.g.
- blood disorders – sore throat, bruising, mouth ulcers
- liver toxicity – nausea, vomiting, abdominal discomfort and dark urine
- respiratory effects – shortness of breath.
  Avoid pregnancy for at least 3 months after stopping.

5) A Acitretin

Acitretin is an oral retinoid used in psoriasis. Should be prescribed by secondary care only. Exclude pregnancy before starting treatment and avoid pregnancy for at least 2 years after stopping. Tazarotene is a topical retinoid for mild/moderate plaque psoriasis. Normal skin must be avoided because of irritation.

6) E Ciclosporin

Ciclosporin should be prescribed by secondary care only. Potent immunosuppressant drug also used in transplantation, atopic dermatitis and rheumatoid arthritis. Be aware of possible drug interactions, including grapefruit juice, which will increase blood levels. Usually used for short-term treatment only, around 8 weeks.

7) F Dithranol

Dithranol's major disadvantages are skin irritation and staining of clothing and skin. It is suitable for application to chronic extensor plaques only, carefully avoiding normal skin. In this way it differs from coal tar.

8) C Calcipotriol

Calcipotriol is a topical vitamin D analogue used in plaque psoriasis. Avoid in patients with calcium metabolism disorders. Does not have the staining or unpleasant smells associated with other topical treatments.

9) J UVA

Psoralens are plant derivatives used with UVA light to increase the effect of irradiation. UV light is associated with premature ageing and skin neoplasms. Combining treatment with other topical therapies can reduce cumulative radiation dose.

10) B Betamethasone

Be aware of the variation in potency of topical steroids to guide prescribing. The *BNF* has a good list for comparison. For example, use of more than 100 g per week of 0.1% betamethasone is likely to cause adrenal suppression. Current evidence suggests that once daily application of steroid creams is likely to be as effective as twice daily.

11) C Non-maleficence

Non-maleficence means 'do no harm'. This most commonly involves scenarios where we avoid giving treatments known to be harmful – here giving a beta-blocker in a patient with asthma.

12) E Confidentiality

Confidentiality is defined as 'ensuring that information is accessible only to those authorized to have access'. Here, as a 15-year-old girl, so long as she is 'Gillick competent', it is acceptable to prescribe contraception; however, it is unlikely that a 'definite guarantee' can ever be given. Knowledge of an abusive relationship for example may prompt a doctor to contact social services. A child can be reassured that any breech of confidentiality can only be carried out in her own best interests or for reasons of public safety.

13) F Justice

Justice, or distributive justice, is the ethical principle that patients who have similar circumstances or conditions should be treated alike. This could apply to two individual patients being treated differently within the same practice, or to whole groups of patients being treated differently in different parts of the country.

14) A Autonomy

Autonomy is a patient's right to make independent decisions and to self-govern. Doctors may not always agree with the wisdom of those decisions.

15) B Beneficence

Beneficence is the basic principle of doing good. Usually referred to alongside the principle of non-maleficence.

16) D Informed consent

Informed consent requires a doctor to tell the patient anything that would substantially affect the patient's decision. This might include the nature or purpose of the treatment, its risks, consequences and alternative courses of action.

Be familiar with these principles and how they might apply to clinical scenarios. Each scenario is likely to involve more than one ethical principle, but it should be possible to prioritize one principle over the others.

17) D Deontology

- *Ethical relativism*: The view that moral values are not absolute but vary with cultures. The rules of current society serve as standard. For example, ethical relativism accepts that cannibalism is acceptable in some cultures, but unacceptable in others.
- *Divine command theory*: Moral values as defined by God. For example, The Ten Commandments.
- *Utilitarianism*: Actions are judged solely by their consequences. Does the end justify the means? For example, in war, a utilitarian view accepts an inevitable loss of life is acceptable to ultimately save more people by bringing down a dictatorship.
- *Deontology*: Moral values defined by rules and duties. These cannot be broken regardless of how to resolve ethical dilemmas. For example, deontology states that it is wrong to steal, even if it is to feed yourself and your hungry family.
- *Virtue ethics*: Emphasizes character rather than rules or consequences. For example, virtue ethics would state that in a negligence case, a doctor with a lazy reputation would be treated more harshly than a doctor with a hard-working reputation.

18) D The number of true negatives detected by the test divided by the true negatives in the population tested

A 60% specificity means that 60% of those who do not have the disease will correctly test negative and the other 40% will test incorrectly positive. Sensitivity is answer E. A 70% sensitivity means that 70% of those with the disease will test positive and the other 30% will test negative.

Sensitivity and specificity are absolute properties of a test. They do not change for a test regardless of how common or uncommon a disease is. They do not necessarily help to decide the clinical usefulness of the test.

The clinical usefulness of a test depends greatly on how common a condition is in the population. The positive and negative predictive values (PPV and NPV) of a test depend on the prevalence of the disease and may vary from population to population. PPV and NPV are therefore better at assessing the clinical usefulness of the test. If a test is uncommon in a population, most positive tests will be false positives, even in a test with a high specificity.

The definitions of sensitivity, specificity, PPV and NPV can be written in a number of different formats as listed below. It is important to understand these definitions are well as possible as there may be multiple questions taking in these concepts:

	Disease +ve	Disease −ve
Test +ve	a (true positives)	b (false positives)
Test −ve	c (false negatives)	d (true negatives)

Sensitivity =
$a/(a+c)$.
The proportion of true positives correctly identified by the test.
True positive tested | Total disease positive.

Specificity =
$d/(b+d)$.
The proportion of true negatives correctly identified by the test.
True negative tested | Total disease negative.

Positive predictive value =
$a/(a+b)$.
The proportion of those who test positive who actually have the disease.
True positives | Total testing positive.

Negative predictive value =
$d/(c+d)$.
The proportion of those who tested negative who do not have the disease.
True negatives | Total testing negative.

19) E It is useful for comparing analgesia treatment for chronic osteoarthritis

In a crossover trial, the patients act as their own control. The subject has one drug or treatment, then a washout period followed by another drug or treatment or placebo. The effect can then be compared within the same individual. It is an inappropriate trial design for use in acute or self-limiting conditions. It is a good study design for chronic conditions. Each patient is a perfectly matched control for him or herself. Because each person is acting as their own control, it is usually possible to use smaller numbers to get the same power. It is just as easy to randomize and double blind as for other study designs. The order in which the treatments are received is randomized.

20) D Guillain–Barré syndrome

Guillain–Barré is an example of acute symmetrical peripheral neuropathy, which can be fatal. Patients may not have absent reflexes in the first few hours of the disease. Treatment with IV immunoglobulin expedites recovery and reduces disability.

21) G Systematic vasculitis

Multiple mononeuropathy in a patient with a connective tissue disorder is most likely due to vasculitis, in particular polyarteritis nodosa (PAN) or Churg–Strauss syndrome. Treatment is with steroids and other immunosuppressants such as cyclophosphamide.

22) B Cisplatin therapy

Both cisplatin therapy and underlying neoplasm are associated with chronic symmetrical peripheral neuropathy. Another consideration would be a spinal cord compression, but a multiple peripheral neuropathy is more likely in this scenario.

23) A Charcot–Marie–Tooth disease

Charcot–Marie–Tooth or peroneal muscular atrophy is an autosomal dominant sensorimotor neurological condition. Features include pes cavus, claw toes and spread from peroneal muscles to upper and lower limbs.

24) C Diabetic neuropathy

Peripheral neuropathy is a common consequence of diabetes. Consider undiagnosed diabetes here. Neuropathies are usually sensory or autonomic in nature, manifesting as pain, impotence or gastric motility disorders.

25) B Case-control study

This study would be done prospectively. The cohort is the group of medical students. The cohort is then followed up to compare outcomes.

26) A Case-control study
Because limb hypoplasia is rare, this study should be done retrospectively. A group of babies with limb hypoplasia are matched to control babies without limb hypoplasia. The two groups are then compared for the exposure of interest, thalidomide treatment in the mother.

27) C Cross-sectional study
This study does not take place over time. A cross-sectional study or point prevalence study takes a snapshot in time of the five GP practices' prescribing habits.

28) D Meta-analysis (Forest plot)
A Forest plot will allow the results from multiple trials asking the same question to be displayed simultaneously to allow comparisons and an overall conclusion to be drawn.

29) C Death due to chronic alcoholism
Notification of death to the Coroner or Procurator Fiscal in Scotland is a common multiple choice question. Deaths to be reported to the Coroner include:
- unexpected deaths, including suspected suicide
- accidents and injuries
- industrial diseases (e.g. asbestosis)
- service disability pensioners
- deaths where the doctor has not attended within the past 14 days
- death arising from abuse
- unknown cause of death
- deaths within a day of hospital admission
- poisoning (though not alcoholism)
- medically related deaths (e.g. anaesthetic or operation complications)
- abortions
- deaths in prison
- stillbirths where there is doubt over whether the baby was born alive. In Scotland, additional reportable deaths to the Procurator Fiscal are deaths in foster children and the newborn.
 In practical terms, all such deaths should be discussed with the Coroner's office; however, a referral does not always result in a post mortem examination. Where a Coroner post mortem is required, family consent is not required. Next of kin consent must be obtained for a hospital post mortem.

30) C Olanzapine
Olanzapine is an atypical antipsychotic drug; risperidone and amisulpride are alternative antipsychotics. These drugs may be better at reducing psychotic symptoms with less extrapyramidal side effects of the older dopamine-blocking drugs such as haloperidol or chlorpromazine. Clozapine is reserved for treatment of refractory schizophrenia and should only be administered in hospital. Piportil depot injections are reserved for patients who are unreliable with oral therapy. Pimozide is not used first line because it requires cardiac monitoring.

31) A Acute myocardial infarction

Acute MI changes are likely familiar to you. Q waves may be present for a number of reasons. Permanent Q waves indicate myocardial necrosis, for example in cardiomyopathy, amyloidosis or sarcoidosis, not just myocardial infarction. Transient Q waves indicate failure of myocardial function without cell death. Causes include hypoxia, coronary arterial spasm, hyperkalaemia or hypothermia.

32) E Pulmonary embolus

These classic changes (S1, Q3, T3) associated with pulmonary embolus (PE) are uncommon but are highly specific for PE. Sinus tachycardia is the commonest ECG feature in PE.

33) D Acute pericarditis

Acute pericarditis presents with sharp central chest pain relieved by leaning forwards. ECG changes would be expected on all leads.

34) B Low potassium levels

In addition to low potassium level, other causes of long QT include congenital, hypocalcaemia, hypomagnesaemia and hypothermia. Drug causes are procainamide, quinidine and amiodarone.

35) C High calcium levels

In addition to a high calcium level, the other cause of shortened QT is digoxin toxicity.

It is wise to revise common ECG changes prior to the AKT. Questions could occur in the form of EGC interpretation or descriptions of ECG changes as above.

36) A Amoxicillin

Note in this question that the child presents 36 hours after onset of symptoms. Acute otitis media (OM) in a child <2 years of age should be treated with antibiotics within 48 hours of onset of signs and symptoms of middle ear inflammation, especially with a temperature of 39°C or greater. Antibiotics are of most benefit in the under twos. Without antibiotics, OM resolves within 24 hours in about 60% of children, and within 3 days in about 80% of children.

Observation is recommended for children over 6 months with an uncertain diagnosis, mild otalgia and temperature <39°C. In children aged 2 years and older, antibiotics are only indicated in severe illness (moderate to severe otalgia or high fever with a certain diagnosis of OM).

37) C Viral gastroenteritis

Notifiable diseases in England and Wales

Acute encephalitis
Anthrax
Cholera
Diphtheria
Dysentery
Enteric fever
Food poisoning
Haemophilus influenzae
Leprosy
Leptospirosis
Malaria
Measles, mumps and rubella
Meningitis (meningococcal
  and pneumococcal)

Ophthalmia neonatorum

Paratyphoid fever
Plague
Poliomyelitis
Relapsing fever
Scarlet fever
Smallpox
Tetanus
Typhus
Tuberculosis
Viral haemorrhagic fever
Viral hepatitis, i.e., hepatitis
  types A, B and C
Viral meningococcal septicaemia
  (without meningitis)
Whooping cough (pertussis)
Yellow fever

Notifiable diseases in Scotland

The list of notifiable diseases in Scotland differs from that in the rest of the UK. The body responsible for national surveillance in Scotland is the Scottish Centre for Infection and Environmental Health (SCIEH).

Not included in Scotland	Included in Scotland
Acute encephalitis	Chickenpox
Cerebrospinal fever	Continued fever
Enteric fever	Erysipelas
Leprosy	Legionellosis
Viral meningococcal septicaemia	Lyme disease
Ophthalmia neonatorum	Puerperal fever
Yellow fever	Rabies
	Toxoplasmosis
	Typhoid fever

When trying to remember these, there are some rules of thumb that might help:
- infections which spread rapidly and are potentially life threatening
- infections not easily treated
- infections, which are on the primary immunization schedule to monitor the effect of immunization
- infections from foreign travel.

38) C Incidents where injury causes 2 days absence from work

Reporting of Injuries, Diseases and Dangerous Occurrences Regulations (RIDDOR) is the mechanism by which the government's Health and Safety Executive monitors industrial injuries. Injured employees must always report details of any accident to be recorded in their employer's accident book. Employers then have to, in turn, report the most serious injuries. Incidents which must be reported to a RIDDOR contact centre include:

- deaths
- major injuries
- over-3-day injuries – where an employee or self-employed person is away from work or unable to perform their normal work duties for more than 3 consecutive days
- injuries to members of the public or people not at work where they are taken from the scene of an accident to hospital
- some work-related diseases
- dangerous occurrences – where something happens that does not result in an injury, but could have done
- CORGI registered gas fitters must also report dangerous gas fittings they find, and gas conveyors/suppliers must report some flammable gas incidents.

39) D Previously failed smoking attempt

A previously failed smoking attempt should not stop a person being encouraged to attempt to quit again. Normally, however, the NHS will not fund a further attempt within 6 months. All of the other answers are relative contraindications to nicotine replacement therapy, which must be balanced with the benefits of stopping smoking. Patches should not be placed onto broken skin of chronic skin conditions. Blood glucose should be monitored closely in diabetic patients. There is not enough evidence currently to warrant co-prescribing nicotine replacement therapy and bupropion (Zyban).

40) C Hyperthyroidism

Hypothyroidism leads to poor hair growth and a coarsening of the hair shaft. The most common cause is fungal scalp infections. In non-scarring alopecia, hair follicles are not damaged and so new hair growth occurs and the follicle openings remain visible. In scarring alopecia, the hair follicles are destroyed. Hair follicle skin markings are lost and hair loss is irreversible. Causes of non-scarring alopecia include alopecia areata, trichotillomania (compulsive pulling of one's hair) and traction alopecia. Scarring alopecia has a more extensive range of causes including common dermatoses such as lichen sclerosus and lichen planus. Skin neoplasms, infections and developmental defects tend to cause scarring alopecia. Scalp ringworm (tinea capitis) may or may not be scarring.

41) D Microaneurysms

Clinical signs of diabetic retinopathy include:

- microaneurysms and dot-and-blot intraretinal haemorrhages
- flame-shaped haemorrhages
- retinal oedema: due to capillary leakage; has a predilection for the macula
- hard exudates: yellow, lipid precipitates which result from resorption of retinal oedema
- cotton wool spots: represent areas of axonal disruption secondary to ischaemia.

Visual loss results mainly from macular oedema, macular ischaemia, vitreous haemorrhage and retinal distortion or detachment.

Diabetic patients should be screened annually. Laser treatment is used to get closure of leaky blood vessels or microaneurysms. Panretinal photocoagulation is used to treat neovascularization.

42) C Arteriovenous nipping

It is not necessary to learn the different grades of hypertensive retinopathy, but understanding the natural history aids in remembering the features present in hypertensive versus diabetic retinopathy:

- Grade 1: Arteriolar attenuation
- Grade 2: Focal arteriolar attenuation with AV nipping (these two signs are a response to hypertension, causing arteriolar spasm and narrowing)
- Grade 3: Haemorrhages, cotton wool spots (due to infarction of the nerve fibre layer of retina)
- Grade 4: Disc swelling – 'malignant' or 'accelerated' phase.

43) E Refer to psychiatric outpatient clinic

44) F Urgent referral for admission

45) B Increase the dose of antidepressant or consider switching to another

Although the law has recently changed in England and Wales regarding the criteria for section under the Mental Health Act, the principles remain the same. Patients who you have reason to believe may have a mental health disorder and are a risk to themselves or others due to this are eligible for section under the relevant Mental Health Act. Any serious but stable clinical situation can wait to be seen at the psychiatric clinic.

46) C Theophylline

Theophylline has a narrow therapeutic margin, so drug level testing and dose adjustment can prevent toxicity. INR (international normalized ratio) is a measure of time to clot against a control. It does not directly measure the blood level of a drug. Other drugs, which require level testing, are gentamicin, vancomycin, digoxin and methotrexate. Other drug levels can be measured in overdose such as salicylic acid and paracetamol.

47) G Helman

48) H Balint

49) D Neighbour

50) B Stott and Davis

51) I Berne

52) C Pendleton et al.

53) F Calgary–Cambridge observation guide

54) A Byrne and Long

Consultation models
Byrne and Long (1976) – Doctors talking to patients: six logical steps to a consultation
    1. Establish a relationship.
    2. Discover the issues.
    3. Verbal and/or physical exam.
    4. Consider the condition.
    5. Detail investigation and treatment.
    6. Consultation terminated, usually by doctor.

Stott and Davis (1979) – The exceptional potential in each primary care consultation
    1. Management of presenting problems.
    2. Modification of help-seeking behaviour.
    3. Management of continuing problems.
    4. Opportunistic health promotion.

Pendleton et al. (1984) – The Consultation: seven tasks
    1. Define the reason for the patient's attendance.
    2. Consider other problems.
    3. Choose appropriate action
    4. Shared understanding with the patient.
    5. Involve the patient in management decisions.
    6. Use time and resources well.
    7. Establish and maintain the doctor–patient relationship.

Neighbour (1987) – The inner consultation: five signposts in a consultation
    1. Connecting.
    2. Summarizing.
    3. Handing over.
    4. Safety netting.
    5. Housekeeping.

Calgary–Cambridge observation guide (1996) – Stages of a consultation

1. Initiating the session.
2. Gathering information.
3. Building the relationship.
4. Explanation and planning.
5. Closing the session.

Tuckett et al. (1985) – The meeting of two experts

The consultation is a meeting between two experts.

1. Doctors are experts in medicine.
2. Patients are experts in their own illnesses
3. Shared understanding is the aim.
4. Doctors should seek to understand the patient's beliefs.
5. Doctors should address explanations in terms of the patient's belief system.

Helman's folk model (1981) – Patient's health beliefs

1. What has happened?
2. Why?
3. Why me?
4. Why now?
5. What if I do nothing?
6. What should I do?

Balint (1957) – The doctor, his patient and the illness: the doctor as a drug

Berne (1964) – Transactional analysis – games people play. Parent, adult and child ego states

55) E Terminal illness

Essential services are those which all practices must carry out. They include day-to-day medical care, care of the terminally ill and chronic disease management. Additional services which carry additional payment include:

- cervical screening
- child health surveillance
- maternity services
- contraceptive services
- vaccinations and immunizations
- maternity services
- minor surgical procedures.

56) B Social deprivation
Factors influencing consultation rates are as follows:

Lower consultation rates	Higher consultation rates
High list size	New patients
Personal lists	Elderly patients
Not prescribing for minor ailments	Social deprivation
Summer months	Winter months
	Practices encouraging health promotion

57) A Information more than 2 years old
The age of the information should not be a barrier to access.
Information regarding a third party is not appropriate to access, unless
that third person is a healthcare professional. Information which may
cause mental or physical harm may be withheld. Information where the
patient is not identified can be withheld. This is one reason why audits
are carried out without using patient identifiers. Where access is sought
to a deceased person's record, access is permissible where disclosure is
required to satisfy a claim relating to the death, e.g. in mesothelioma.

58) D Repeated refusal of a patient to accept a GP's advice
Patients have the right to not accept a GP's advice. Patients continuing to
smoke is a good example of this. Difference of opinion is not a reason
for removal from the practice list. Justification for removal from a
practice list includes deception for the purposes of fraud, residence
outwith the practice area and verbal or physical violence. If a person is
removed from the practice list, it is usual for other members of the same
household to be removed also, though this is not universal.

59) E Responsibility for minimizing radiation exposure lies both with the
referrer and with the radiographer or radiologist carrying out the
imaging.

60) D Atlanto-axial subluxation in a patient with rheumatoid arthritis prior
to a general anaesthetic
Subluxation of the atlanto-axial joint can occur in rheumatoid arthritis
or in Down's syndrome. When considering the safety of a general
anaesthetic, flexion–extension views are carried out to assess the safety
of intubation for general anaesthetic. If not carried out in general
practice, it would be carried out as part of an anaesthetic assessment.
Neither dizziness nor torticollis is an indication for X-ray on its own as
there are no causes that would show up on X-ray. Cervical rib, a
congenital additional rib arising from C7, should be diagnosed from a
chest X-ray. Degenerative change on its own is not an indication for X-
ray as the diagnosis should be clinical although lots of these X-rays are
done in practice.

61) B Hinduism

People of any faith or culture will vary in how they carry out customs. It is important to discuss relevant issues with individual patients.

62) B Right middle ear

In vestibular neuronitis, nystagmus is more pronounced on looking away from the lesion. Nystagmus arising from the brain stem or cerebellum causes a multi-directional (rather than horizontal) nystagmus. This does not resolve on looking straight ahead.

63) B 10 mg diazepam

Benzodiazepines should only be prescribed short term to prevent dependence. When initiating a withdrawal plan, the dose should be converted to diazepam at night, which will act to help insomnia at night and anxiety during the day. This can then be gradually reduced. Approximate equivalent doses of 5 mg diazepam are:
- 15 mg chlordiazepoxide
- 0.5–1 mg loprazolam
- 500 mcg lorazepam
- 0.5–1 mg lormetazepam
- 5 mg nitrazepam
- 15 mg oxazepam
- 10 mg temazepam.

64) C $\frac{1}{2}$ total 24-hour oral morphine dose

An intramuscular or subcutaneous dose of morphine is half the total oral dose. The dose is then either divided by 6 to be given every 4 hours or infused over 24 hours using a subcutaneous pump. Where diamorphine is being used parenterally, the dose is one-third of the total oral morphine dose.

65) B Leflunomide

Leflunomide is a new disease-modifying drug (DMD) for the treatment of rheumatoid arthritis. It is very popular in the US and is now available on NHS prescription. Patient's BP and serum LFTs should be monitored. An alternative NSAID would be inappropriate. Ciclosporin tends to be used when other DMDs are not appropriate. Blood monitoring is required for all DMDs used in rheumatoid arthritis. The tumour necrosis factor inhibitors (TNF-α) adalimumab, etanercept and infliximab would also be options but are ideally used alongside methotrexate. All of these treatments should be initiated by secondary care.

66) C FEVI/FVC < 0.7

67) E FEVI/FVC > 0.7

68) D Access compliance and inhaler technique

69) B Continue treatment

70) A Further investigation

71) B Continue treatment

72) D Study D
Study D is the only study to show a statistically significant benefit, because the confidence interval line does not cross the line of no difference. 'I' represents an odds ratio of I, i.e. no difference.

73) C Study C
Study C has reached statistical significance showing evidence of harm. Study A has also done this but its mean is lower. It has also been a smaller study.

74) D Study D
The area of the black square denotes the power of the trial given to the meta-analysis. Study D has the largest square.

75) E Study E
The length of the line emerging from the square represents the confidence intervals.

76) F I
Only one of the studies shows a statistically significant benefit, i.e. only one study showed a positive effect where the confidence interval range did not cross the line of no difference.

77) K Meta-analysis shows overall benefit
The diamond at the bottom of the graph represents the statistical combination of all of the previous studies. Although only one study showed a statistically significant benefit, it was sufficiently powered to negate the harmful findings of the other studies.

Forest plots are used in meta-analyses to summarize data from multiple studies. They comprise a central square with lengths of horizontal lines emerging from them. The size of the squares represents the weight that the individual study contributed to the meta-analysis. The length of the lines represents the confidence intervals, though not always 95% confidence intervals. In general, the larger the study, the narrower the confidence interval and the larger the square. It then follows that the studies with the largest squares will tend to have the smallest confidence intervals.

The overall estimate from the metaanalysis and its confidence interval are put at the bottom, represented as a diamond. The centre of the diamond represents the pooled point estimate, and its horizontal tips represent the confidence interval. Significance is achieved at the set level if the diamond is clear of the line of no effect.

Interpretation of study graphs is likely to form AKT questions. Be sure you are familiar with their use.

78) D Storing a locked bag in the boot of a locked car

A doctor's bag must be lockable. If it is in the car, it should be locked and out of sight. Simply having the car locked is not a high enough level of security. The bag should also be locked inside the car. Some doctors prefer to have a separate bag for drugs for this reason. Diagnostic equipment can be carried into a house in an unlocked bag, while the drugs remain locked in the car unless needed. Other considerations for a doctor's bag containing drugs are as follows:

- do not leave the bag unattended during house visits
- avoid extremes of temperature
- drugs given from the doctor's bag should be in a suitable container, properly labelled with patient and prescription details
- check drugs twice yearly to ensure they are still in date.

79) E Papillary

The order of frequency of thyroid cancers can be remembered via the mnemonic 'Presents For My Lovely Aunt':

- Papillary
- Follicular
- Medullary
- Lymphoma
- Anaplastic

Age ranges for these types of thyroid cancer are:

- Papillary: 10–40 yrs
- Follicular: 40–60 yrs
- Medullary: occurs at any age
- Lymphoid: occurs at any age; may be primary or secondary
- Anaplastic: 50–60 yrs.

Anaplastic carcinoma is the most aggressive tumour, whereas papillary carcinoma is a lower grade malignancy with significant metastatic potential. Also bear in mind the possibility of secondary tumour from breast, kidney, lung or colorectal tumours.

80) D Lewy body dementia

This man has symptoms of Parkinsonism along with hallucinations and delusions. This pattern fits with a diagnosis of Lewy body dementia.

Progressive supranuclear palsy (Steele–Richardson syndrome) presents with features of Parkinsonism with ophthalmoplegia and dementia. Multi-system atrophy refers to a number of conditions characterized by Parkinsonism, autonomic symptoms and cerebellar and pyramidal features. Features of Parkinsonism may be found in longstanding sufferers of schizophrenia due to long-term use of dopamine-blocking antipsychotic drugs.

81) A The ability to be talked or calmed out of a seizure
Seizure diagnosis is complex and so the diagnosis of factitious seizures should not be made lightly. Seizures only when people are present may be suggestive, though not diagnostic. There may be preserved consciousness in frontal lobe seizures. There may be speech in complex partial seizures. If factitious seizures are suspected, share this suspicion with secondary care. Video telemetry is the most reliable way to make the diagnosis.

82) E Subdural haematoma
The elderly are at particular risk of subdural haematoma. The level of trauma may have been minor and not recognized by the patient. Subdural haematoma in the elderly can have a subacute or even chronic presentation with increasing confusion, mild hemiparesis and seizures. It may mimic dementia, stroke or malignancy.

83) C Carbamazepine
Many drugs have an effect on liver enzymes. If a drug is a liver enzyme inducer, it will increase the rate of metabolism of certain drugs. A mnemonic to remember the drugs which cause liver enzyme induction is PC BRAS: Phenytoin, Carbamazepine, Barbiturates, Rifampicin, Alcoholism, Sulphonylureas.

84) A Erythromycin
Rifampicin is a liver enzyme inducer and so may reduce INR. Erythromycin is a liver enzyme inhibitor. These may be remembered by the mnemonic ODEVICES: Omeprazole, Disulfiram, Erythromycin, Valproate, Isoniazid, Cimetidine, Ciprofloxacin, Ethanol (acutely) and Sulphonamides. The drugs most used in clinical practice to be affected by this process are warfarin, phenytoin, theophyllines and the oral contraceptive pill.

85) C Change felodipine to an ACE inhibitor
Calcium channel blockers may be associated with gravitational oedema. Bendroflumethiazide would normally be the next choice in a 70 year old, but given the rheumatic disease and indometacin being excreted by the kidneys, an ACE inhibitor would be more appropriate.

86) G One test $\geq$ 11.1 mmol/l

87) C One test $\geq$ 7.0 mmol/l

88) D Two tests $\geq$ 7.0 mmol/l

89) G One test $\geq$ 11.1 mmol/l

90) H Two tests $\geq$ 11.1 mmol/l

91) E One test $\geq$ 7.8 mmol/l
This question looks very difficult at first! You should, however, be familiar with glucose testing and the diagnosis of diabetes and impaired glucose tolerance. Interpretation of diabetes diagnosis is common.
Diagnosing diabetes
- Oral glucose tolerance testing:
  - $\geq$11.1 mmol/l, the patient is diabetic
  - $\geq$7.8 and <11.1 mmol/l is impaired glucose tolerance
  - <7.8 mmol/l, the patient is not diabetic
- Random glucose:
  - if symptomatic, one random glucose $\geq$11.1 mmol/l
  - if asymptomatic, two random glucose $\geq$11.1 mmol/l
- Fasting glucose:
  - if symptomatic, one fasting glucose $\geq$7.0 mmol/l
  - if asymptomatic, two fasting glucose $\geq$7.0 mmol/l
- Impaired fasting glycaemia
  - fasting glucose $\geq$ 6.1 mmol/l and <7 mmol/l: do an oral glucose tolerance test to clarify the diagnosis.

92) D BMI > 30

93) C BMI > 28

94) D BMI > 30

95) B BMI > 27

96) F BMI > 40

97) E BMI > 35

98) G BMI > 50
BMI figures are the best statistics to memorize. Diabetes and hypertension indicate increased cardiovascular risk, requiring more aggressive treatment of obesity. The guidelines to treating obesity are as

follows:

- *Step 1* – Lifestyle measures: These must form the cornerstone of all obesity treatments.
- *Step 2* – Drug treatment: Continue treatment beyond 3 months if a patient has successfully lost >5% of their original bodyweight. Continue beyond 12 months only after discussing ongoing risks and benefits. Orlistat should not be continued beyond 24 months. Sibutramine treatment should not be continued beyond 12 months. Sibutramine requires monitoring of blood pressure.
- *Step 3* – Bariatric surgery: Although the NICE guidelines above apply, variations in availability throughout the country means local referral guidelines may vary.
  Waist circumference is also a useful assessor of cardiovascular risk conferred by obesity and can be used to guide treatment:
- *In men*: Waist circumference 94–102 cm is high; >102 cm is very high.
- *In women*: Waist circumference 80–88 cm is high; >88 cm is very high.

99) A FSH

An FSH level >30 IU/L with amenorrhoea is diagnostic of the menopause. The risks and benefits of HRT are still a cause for debate. HRT is generally recommended for a maximum of 5 years. As stopping HRT suddenly can cause a rebound in menopausal symptoms, it should be phased out over around 6 months. HRT should only be prescribed for distressing menopausal symptoms. HRT confers no cardiovascular protection as has been suggested in the past.

100) B Over-exercising

Excess exercise causes suppression of gonadotrophin-releasing hormone (GnRH), which in turn causes amenorrhoea. The exact mechanism of the hormonal change is unknown. Female athletes are also at risk of osteoporosis and eating disorders. Pregnancy should be associated with other symptoms and abdominal swelling, though concealed pregnancy is a potential cause of unexplained amenorrhoea. Premature ovarian failure would be accompanied by menopausal symptoms. Polycystic ovarian syndrome is associated with hirsutism and obesity, though these features are not universal.

AKT Paper 2: Questions

1) *Stroke thrombolysis*

   You receive a phone call from the husband of a 69-year-old previously healthy lady. He is panicking because he says she cannot talk properly. Her face is drooping to one side and he cannot get her to stand up out of her armchair. 1 hour ago she was completely normal. You call an ambulance and page the on-call stroke physician to discuss.

   What is the maximum safe window for thrombolysis in thrombotic stroke?

   A 2 hours
   B 3 hours
   C 6 hours
   D 12 hours
   E 24 hours

2) *Clinical governance*

   Elements of clinical governance include all of the following EXCEPT:

   A Clinical audit
   B Detection of adverse events
   C Leadership
   D Responsibility lying with clinical rather than non-clinical staff
   E Professional development programmes

3) *Peripheral vascular disease*

   A 57-year-old male patient with known angina complains of calf pain on walking 50 m.

   Which of the following is most likely to improve his walking distance?

   A Walking
   B Aspirin
   C Statin
   D Lowering his blood pressure to <140/85
   E ACE inhibitor
   F Cilostazol

4–8) *Missed contraception*

For the following situations, establish whether the patient is currently 'protected' or 'unprotected' by their contraception according to guidance in the *BNF*:

A Protected. No additional contraception required
B Unprotected. Additional contraception required for 7 days

4) A 23-year-old woman presents 24 hours after sex. She has missed yesterday's pill from her packet of Microgynon 30. She has now taken yesterday's pill and today's pill. She is on day 17 of her packet.

5) A 27-year-old woman phones for advice. She is taking Loestrin 20. She has missed 2 days worth of pills and is enquiring about additional contraception. She is on day 8 of her packet.

6) A 45-year-old woman is using the contraceptive patch. It fell off during the night. The maximum time it may have been off is 12 hours. The patch has been reapplied and is sticking well.

7) A 20-year-old woman has missed three of her Microgynon 30 pills. She is in her second week of the pack.

8) An 18-year-old woman is having her Depo-Provera injection 12 weeks and 3 days after her previous injection.

9–12) *Hepatitis B serology*

For the following set of hepatitis B serology results, which is the most appropriate interpretation?

A Immune, post-vaccination
B Immune, past exposure to HBV
C Infected, low risk of transmission
D Infected, high risk of transmission

9) sAb +ve: sAg −ve/cAb −ve/eAg −ve/eAb −ve/DNA −ve

10) sAb −ve: sAg +ve/cAb +ve/eAg +ve/eAb −ve/DNA +ve

11) sAb −ve: sAg +ve/cAb +ve/eAg −ve/eAb +ve/DNA −ve

12) sAb +ve: sAg −ve/cAb +ve/eAg −ve/eAb +ve/DNA −ve

13) *Summarizing data*

Your practice has carried out a study of random blood glucose levels within your practice population. You are asked to write up the results. The plotted data create a skewed graph. They should therefore be summarized by stating:

A The median and range
B The median and standard deviation
C The mean and standard deviation
D The mean and range
E The mean and 95% confidence intervals

14) *Cohort studies*

Which ONE of the following is true regarding cohort studies?

A Cohort studies are retrospective
B Cohort studies are better than other study designs for measuring the incidence of a disease in the population
C Cohort studies are better than other study designs for measuring the prevalence of a disease in the population
D Cohort studies can only be used to compare two groups with each other
E A cohort study is a good design to use when looking at a rare outcome

15) *Standard deviations*

When looking at study data summarized as mean and standard deviation, what percentage of data lies within mean ± 2 standard deviations?

A 68%
B 88%
C 95%
D 98%
E 99%

16) *Standard error of the mean*

Standard error of the mean (SEM) is:

A SEM $=$ standard deviation^2
B SEM $=$ standard deviation$/\sqrt{n}$
C SEM $=$ $\sqrt{\text{variance}}$
D SEM $=$ variance^2
E SEM $=$ standard deviation$/\sqrt{\text{variance}}$

17–20) *Drugs used in breast cancer treatment*

A 45-year-old woman attends your surgery for pain relief as she is recovering from a mastectomy and axillary node clearance for breast cancer. She is awaiting her pathology results and further advice from the hospital about which treatment to start next. She attends with lots of articles from the Internet and wants to know what all these drugs are.

Match each drug name with its mode of action:

A Oestrogen receptor antagonists
B Aromatase inhibitors
C Monoclonal antibodies against overexpression of HER2/neu oncogene
D Cytotoxic chemotherapeutic agents

17) Anastrozole (Arimidex)

18) Trastuzumab (Herceptin)

19) Docetaxel, doxorubicin and cyclophosphamide

20) Tamoxifen

21–24) *Medical treatments in Parkinson's disease*

A 55-year-old patient presents with dropping her car keys and a feeling of unsteadiness on her feet. This has deteriorated over the past 6 months. On examination she has a resting pill-rolling tremor, cogwheel rigidity and a mildly shuffling gait. You diagnose Parkinson's disease and refer her to the local Parkinson's specialist physician.

Match each of the following medications with their class:

A Beta-blockers
B Dopamine receptor (D2) agonists
C L-Dopa
D Catechol-O-methyltransferase inhibitors
E Monoamine oxidase-B inhibitors
F Antimuscarinic drugs

21) Entacapone and tolcapone

22) Benzatropine, orphenadrine, procyclidine and trihexyphenidyl/benhexol

23) Bromocriptine, apomorphine, cabergoline, pergolide, pramipexole, ropinirole and rotigotine

24) Selegiline, rasagiline

25–31) *Fitness to drive*
   Match the following scenarios with the appropriate fitness-to-drive regulations:

   A No driving licence restrictions
   B 1 month off driving
   C 6 months off driving
   D 12 months off driving
   E Disqualified from driving until treated
   F Permanently barred and requires DVLA notification
   G Refusal or revocation
   H Driving must cease until cause identified
   I Relicensing when symptom-free for 6/52

25) A man reaches his 70th birthday and is fit and well.

26) A 50-year-old public transport bus driver has a persistent blood pressure of 180/100 mmHg.

27) A 60-year-old man is diagnosed with metastatic carcinoma of the lung with secondaries in the bone and brain.

28) A 47-year-old man has been diagnosed with obstructive sleep apnoea. He has suffered from daytime sleepiness for a number of years.

29) A 30-year-old man has colour blindness and a visual acuity of 6/9 in both eyes.

30) A 20-year-old IVDA heroin misuser tests positive for opiates in his urine. He would like to initiate methadone treatment.

31) A 35-year-old HGV driver reports that he faints at the sight of blood.

32) *Stroke presentation*
The single most common presentation of stroke is:

A Aphasia
B Dysphagia
C Loss of consciousness
D Sudden onset of hemiplegia
E Sudden visual field deficit

33) *BP targets in secondary prevention*
A 56-year-old male patient attends your surgery 2 months after having had a heart attack. He is very grateful for your prompt diagnosis and is serious about reducing his risk of having further problems. He asks what his target should be in reducing his blood pressure. He is not diabetic.
What according to NICE guidance for secondary prevention of MI is his BP target?

A <180/110
B <140/85
C <140/90
D <130/80
E <125/75

34) *BP targets*
A 45-year-old surgical nurse is diagnosed with primary hypertension with a BP 165/97. She is started on an ACE inhibitor and starts to modify her lifestyle with diet and exercise. She also has diet-controlled type II diabetes. She has no history of heart or kidney disease.
She buys a home BP monitor and wants to know what BP target she should be aiming for. Your practice protocol works to NICE guidance.

A <160/100
B <140/90
C <140/80
D <135/75
E <125/75

35–36) *Quality and Outcomes Framework BP targets*
You are auditing your practice management of hypertension. Your practice manager suggests that Quality and Outcomes Framework (QOF) targets are used as audit standards.
For the following circumstances, what is the QOF target?

A <160/100
B <150/80
C <145/85
D <135/75
E <125/75

35) A patient with no history of heart disease, diabetes or kidney disease?

36) A diabetic patient?

37) *Drugs causing gout*
A 60-year-old farmer presents with acute pain at the base of his big toe. He is diagnosed with gout. You review his medication list to establish if any of his medications might have caused the attack.
All of the following are causes of gout EXCEPT:

A Aspirin
B Ciclosporin
C Ethambutol
D Diclofenac
E Nicotinic acid

38) *Liver disease*
A 20-year-old man comes to your surgery worried he has liver disease. He says his eyes sometimes become a bit yellow, especially if he is run down or has been ill. There is no change to his urine or stool colour. He is otherwise fit and well, running half marathons in his spare time. He drinks two cans of lager per week. His Mum and Dad say that he has always been this way, with his skin having a yellow tinge to it during childhood illnesses. His Dad has the same symptoms but has never seen a doctor about it. On examination his liver is non-tender and of normal size. He has no other physical abnormalities and no evidence of jaundice at present. His fasting liver function tests show an isolated raised bilirubin.
What is the most likely diagnosis here?

A Wilson's disease
B Haemochromatosis
C Gilbert's syndrome
D Alcoholic liver disease
E Budd–Chiari syndrome

39–43) *Stages of change model*

When considering a patient's attempts to make lifestyle changes, complete the following algorithm to describe the stages of change:

A Post-contemplation
B Contemplation
C Maintenance
D Action
E Relapse
F Decision

The cycle of change

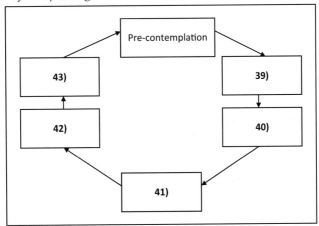

44) *The gold standards framework in community palliative care*

You wish to improve how your practice deals with end of life care. You wish to set up a palliative care register.

Which of the following is NOT one of the 7Cs, or key tasks of the Palliative Care Gold Standards Framework?

A Counselling
B Communication
C Coordination of care
D Control of symptoms
E Continuity including out of hours

45–49) *Childhood illnesses*

For each of the patients below select the single most likely diagnosis.

A Appendicitis
B Bronchiolitis
C Gastroenteritis
D Hand, foot and mouth disease
E Henoch–Schönlein purpura
F Kawasaki's disease
G Meningococcal septicaemia
H Pneumonia

45) A 13-year-old girl presents with a non-blanching rash and drowsiness.

46) A 10-year-old boy presents with a haemorrhagic purpuric rash over the lower half of his body.

47) An 18-month-old baby presents with fever and vomiting. The ears, throat and chest exams are normal.

48) A 2-month-old baby presents with wheeze and cough. On examination, basal crepitations are present.

49) A 3-year-old girl presents with spiking fever, dry cough, left shoulder tip pain and left upper abdominal pain.

50–53) *Pendleton's rules for feedback*
As part of an appraisal, you are observing consultation videos of your practice colleagues. Put the following Pendleton's rules for feedback in the correct order:

A Observers can make negative remarks
B Performer can make negative remarks
C Observers can make positive remarks
D Performer can make positive remarks

50) First event:

51) Second event:

52) Third event:

53) Fourth event:

54) *Occupational disease*

A 56-year-old male patient has recently been diagnosed with lung carcinoma. He wonders whether his previous job in a construction company may have contributed.

Which of the following occupational exposures is associated with increased risk of lung cancer?

A Blue asbestos (Crocidolite) exposure from the construction industry
B Cadmium exposure from working in a battery factory
C Fungal α-amylase exposure from a commercial baker
D Vinyl chloride exposure in a PVC factory
E Wood dust in a furniture factory

55) *Contraindictions to MRI*

A 34-year-old man has a football injury, which has failed to settle over 12 weeks. You suspect a medial meniscal tear. You wish to send him for an MRI scan.

Which of the following is most likely to be a contraindication to MRI?

A Hip screw from a previous fracture
B Cochlear implant
C Claustrophobia
D Tattoos on his ankle
E Umbilical piercing

56) *Lumbar spine X-ray*

A 19-year-old woman attends your surgery with first onset back pain. She is not aware of having injured herself. You decide that her young age warrants a lumbar spine X-ray.

What additional information should you give her?

A Contraception should be used for a week following a lumbar spine X-ray
B The X-ray should not be carried out during her period
C The X-ray should not be carried out after day 10 of her cycle
D She should bring a negative pregnancy test to show to the radiographer
E The X-ray can be carried out at any point in her period so long as she is sure she is not pregnant

57–71) *Pedigree charts*

For the symbols below, match their meaning within a genetic pedigree diagram from the following list.

A Adopted child
B Carrier for trait
C Carrier who will never manifest the disease (e.g. in X-linked recessive disease)
D Clinically affected individual
E Consanguinity
F Consultand/Index case
G Deceased individual
H Dizygotic twins
I Female
J Male
K Monozygotic twins
L Partners now separated
M Sex unknown
N Spontaneous abortion
O Termination of pregnancy

Symbols used in pedigree charts

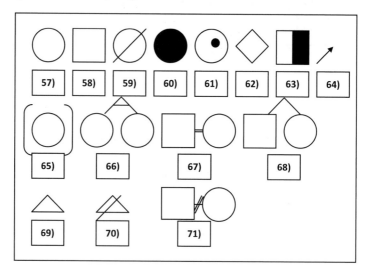

72) *Faith considerations*

Below is a list of considerations which may apply regarding health-care. To which of the following World Faiths might these apply?

• Food is required to be kosher.
• It is considered respectful for a body following death, never to be left alone or in the dark before burial.

- For medication which is required to be taken every day, preparation may be required to prevent the breaking of the Sabbath, as preparing medication may be considered unacceptable work to be carried out on the Sabbath.
- Post mortems may be unacceptable and considered to be desecration of the body.

A Buddhism
B Hinduism
C Islam
D Judaism
E Sikhism

73) *Rinne's test*
A 67-year-old gentleman complains of gradual hearing loss in his left ear. He can hear most things but finds he struggles to hear conversations sometimes in company.
You perform Rinne's test, which is negative, i.e. the tone is better heard through bone than air. This implies:

A Left-sided conductive hearing loss
B Left-sided sensorineural hearing loss
C Right-sided conductive hearing loss
D Right-sided sensorineural hearing loss
E No evidence of hearing loss

74) *Weber's test*
A 67-year-old gentleman complains of gradual hearing loss in his left ear.
You perform Weber's test, which localizes to his left ear. This implies:

A Left-sided conductive hearing loss
B Left-sided sensorineural hearing loss
C Right-sided conductive hearing loss
D Right-sided sensorineural hearing loss
E No evidence of hearing loss

75) *Wilson-Junger screening criteria*
Which of the following is a requirement when devising a screening programme?

A Condition should be life threatening
B Condition should be one that affects all sections of the population
C Screening programme should be agreed nationally
D Screening programme should be 'opt out' in nature
E There should be benefit in starting treatment early

76) *Asthma diagnosis in children*

A 4-year-old boy presents with his mother. He has a history of cough.

Which of the following features makes asthma a more likely diagnosis?

A Symptoms occur only during an upper respiratory tract infection
B Cough without wheeze or difficulty breathing
C History of moist cough
D Family history of atopy
E No wheeze on clinical examination

77) *Asthma*

A 4-year-old boy presents with his mother. He has a history of cough and wheeze but is systemically and developmentally well. Having taken a more detailed history, it is unclear whether his symptoms are due to asthma.

Which is the most INAPPROPRIATE course of action?

A Monitor for other possible causes for the symptoms
B Trial of treatment
C Watchful waiting
D Admit to hospital for investigation
E Carry out spirometry and reversibility testing

78) *Asthma treatment*

A 6-year-old boy presents with his mother. He was diagnosed with asthma 2 years ago and takes a salbutamol inhaler. His mother reports that he is using his inhaler much more frequently than usual. In particular he has been coughing at night. On examination, his chest is clear at present, but his peak flow is reduced to 70% of his best.

Which is the next most appropriate step?

A Add inhaled steroid 200 mcg/day
B Add inhaled steroid 800 mcg/day
C Add inhaled steroid 1000 mcg/day
D Add inhaled steroid 2000 mcg/day
E Add oral leukotriene receptor antagonist

79–83) *Interpretation of funnel plots*

The funnel plot below shows the results of a meta-analysis of trials of a new drug. Each circle represents a different study in the meta-analysis. Interpret the graph to answer the following questions:

A Study a
B Study b
C Study c
D Study d
E Study e
F Study f
G Study g
H 1
I 2
J 3
K 4
L 5
M 6
N 7
O Meta-analysis shows harm
P Meta-analysis shows benefit
Q Meta-analysis shows no statistical difference

Funnel plot

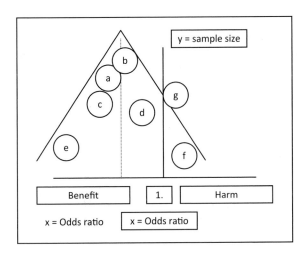

79) Which study claims the most benefit?

80) Which was the smallest study in the meta-analysis?

81) Which study is the clearest outlier?

82) How many studies show a statistically significant benefit with the drug?

83) What is the overall outcome of the analysis?

84) *Confidentiality*
In which of the following situations might confidentiality NOT be ethically and legitimately broken without patient consent?

A   Where there has been an adverse drug reaction
B   When required by court
C   Where there is a risk to public health
D   Where a patient is being cared for in a residential home
E   Where there has been a complaint resulting in a GMC hearing

85) *Entitlement to free treatment on the NHS*
Which of the following is entitled to full free NHS treatment via a GP?

A   A French citizen on holiday in the UK who would like some extra emollient treatment prescribed for his chronic eczema
B   An American citizen who is in the UK for a 6-week working holiday in a UK primary school
C   An Irish citizen who would like a refill of his analgesia prescription
D   A Chinese citizen who has been in the UK for 3 weeks. He has applied for asylum
E   A British citizen who has emigrated to Australia. He returns to the UK every 6 months to visit family. He intends to return to the UK after working for around 5 years

86) *Entitlement to free NHS care*
Which of the following would NOT necessarily be given free on the NHS to an overseas visitor to the UK?

A   Services provided by an Accident and Emergency department
B   Treatment for tuberculosis diagnosed in the UK
C   Treatment for HIV diagnosed while in the UK
D   Treatment for HIV diagnosed abroad but which requires ongoing treatment
E   Family planning services

87) *Urgent referral to colorectal clinic*
Which of the following is NOT an indication for urgent referral to the colorectal clinic with suspected colorectal carcinoma?

A An easily palpable mass in the left iliac fossa and change in bowel habit
B Age over 40 and persistently changed bowel habit with rectal bleeding for over 6 weeks
C Man with unexplained iron deficiency anaemia with an Hb 11 g/100 mL
D Non-menstruating female with unexplained iron deficiency anaemia with an Hb 10 g/100 mL
E Longstanding bowel symptoms with alternating loose stools and constipation

88) *Corticosteroid therapy*
A 67-year-old woman with polymyalgia rheumatica is about to start taking long-term corticosteroid therapy to treat it.
What additional advice should she be given?

A She should have an outpatient DEXA scan to assess her bone density
B She should immediately start bone protection such as alendronate
C Advise her to take a high calcium diet and to exercise regularly
D Start her on bone protective hormone replacement therapy
E She should start on gastric protective omeprazole

89) *Dexamethasone suppression test*
A 33-year-old woman attends complaining of lethargy and weight gain over the past year. She is has a BMI of 40 with acne and striae across her abdomen. Her blood pressure is 165/98. A 48-hour dexamethasone suppression test was performed. Retesting her blood 2 days later showed a cortisol reduction of 50% (failure to suppress adequately).
This would suggest:

A Normal
B Cushing's disease
C Addison's disease
D Type II diabetes
E Cushing's syndrome

90) *Nasal polyps*
A 28-year-old man attends your surgery complaining of longstanding nasal symptoms. He has tried over-the-counter antihistamines but they have been of no help. On examination, moderately sized nasal polyps are present.
Which is the most appropriate initial treatment?

A Beclometasone nasal spray
B Betametasone nasal drops
C Oral prednisolone
D Referral for surgery
E Nasal corticosteroids

91) *Chickenpox*

A 30-year-old pregnant patient presents concerned as her daughter has developed chickenpox. She is 15 weeks pregnant. She has never had chickenpox herself. Her urgent varicella zoster IgG test is negative.

What is the appropriate next step?

A Reassure her no further action is necessary; there is no risk to her pregnancy
B Prescribe oral aciclovir
C Refer for intravenous immunoglobulin
D Refer for intravenous aciclovir
E Refer for termination of pregnancy

92–97) *Cranial nerve lesions*

For each of the following clinical scenarios, match the affected cranial nerve:

A Cranial nerve I
B Cranial nerve II
C Cranial nerve III
D Cranial nerve IV
E Cranial nerve V
F Cranial nerve VI
G Cranial nerve VII
H Cranial nerve VIII
I Cranial nerve IX
J Cranial nerve X
K Cranial nerve XI
L Cranial nerve XII

92) A 76-year-old man complains of inability to smell. He has been referred to Ear, Nose and Throat and no abnormality was found on investigation. He is otherwise well

93) A 50-year-old man presents complaining of double vision. On examination, he has double vision when he looks down and in. He finds this is not as bad if he tilts his head. He suffered a head injury while on a night out a week ago.

94) A 23-year-old woman attends complaining of a blurring of the centre of her vision. This occurs intermittently and affects her left eye. On examination, the optic disc in her left eye appears swollen.

95) A 50-year-old man presents with a right-sided ptosis. On examination his pupil is large and his right eye is turned downwards and out.

96) A 50-year-old man presents complaining of double vision. On examination his double vision occurs on looking outwards.

97) A 45-year-old woman is diagnosed with acoustic neuroma.

98) *Viral upper respiratory tract infection*
A 17-year-old woman attends your surgery complaining of 5 days of cough and sneezing. She has a runny nose and is feeling generally unwell. She has not taken any time off work as she feels it may risk her job. On examination she has a red nose, erythematous throat and her chest is clear.
What is the most likely diagnosis?

A Malingering
B Pneumonia
C Rhinovirus infection
D Streptococcal sore throat
E Allergic rhinitis

99) *Depression in the elderly*
You visit an 80-year-old lady in a residential care home whom the staff think might be depressed.
If treating this lady for depression, which would be the most APPROPRIATE first line treatment?

A Donepezil
B Dosulepin
C Moclobemide
D Sertraline
E Venlafaxine

100) *Insomnia*

A 45-year-old businessman attends your surgery complaining of longstanding poor sleep. He says he has no problem with mood, but has always found his 'head is full of motors' at night and he struggles to get to sleep. He has an important presentation in 2 weeks and feels he needs to be well rested and well prepared. He asks for advice on how he might be able to improve his sleep pattern during this stressful time.

Which of the following pieces of advice is INAPPROPRIATE?

A Don't go to bed until you feel sleepy
B Avoid alcohol in the evening
C A relaxation CD may be helpful
D Short term (up to I week) of low dose nitrazepam running up to his presentation is appropriate in such a stressful circumstance
E Don't stay in bed if you are not asleep

AKT Paper 2: Answers

1) B 3 hours

   Thrombolysis is now well established to be a safe treatment up to 3 hours from onset of symptoms. Fast access CT, to confirm thrombotic stroke and exclude haemorrhage, is becoming more widely available. If the symptoms have resolved, the patient should be referred to the stroke clinic. Patients not on anticoagulation should start antiplatelet therapy: aspirin 50–300 mg daily, or clopidogrel, or a combination of low-dose aspirin and dipyridamole modified release (MR). If patients are aspirin intolerant, an alternative antiplatelet agent, e.g. clopidogrel 75 mg or dipyridamole MR 200 mg twice daily should be used. Note, a combination of aspirin and clopidogrel is not appropriate

2) D Responsibility lying with clinical rather than non-clinical staff

   Clinical governance has a whole section dedicated to it in the curriculum. It is the responsibility of both clinical and non-clinical staff. Elements of clinical governance include:
   - quality improvement (including clinical audit)
   - risk management (including complaints, infection control)
   - staff management (including recruitment, workforce planning and appraisals)
   - leadership
   - planning (including planning for capacity, and cultural aspects)
   - education and training
   - clinical effectiveness (including clinical audit)
   - information management (including record keeping)
   - teamworking.

3) A Walking

   Walking three times per week will produce collateral circulation and help improve walking distance. In addition, cilostazol can help by acting as a peripheral vasodilator. Patients can undergo a 3-month trial of this as a second line therapy. Intermittent claudication should be treated as angina and cardiovascular risk should be aggressively managed. Patients with peripheral vascular disease are at high risk of sudden death

4) A Protected

5) B Unprotected

6) A Protected

7) B Unprotected

8) A Protected

Pill rules:

If one or two 30–35 μg *or* one 20 μg ethinylestradiol pills have been missed, no additional or emergency contraception required. If three or more 30–35 μg *or* two or more 20 μg ethinylestradiol pills have been missed, use condoms/abstain from sex until pills have been taken for 7 days in a row. If missed in week 1, consider emergency contraception if the woman had unprotected sex in the pill-free period or week 1. If missed in week 3, advise to finish the pills in the current pack and start a new pack the next day, omitting the pill-free period.

Regarding the contraceptive patch:

One patch is to be applied once weekly for 3 weeks followed by a patch-free week. If the patch falls off for <24 hours or a patch change is delayed for <48 hours, reapply the patch immediately and continue the cycle. If the patch falls off for >24 hours or if patch change is delayed for >48 hours, start a new cycle. Use additional contraception for 7 days.

Regarding Depo-Provera:

An injection is effective immediately if given <12 weeks and 5 days after the previous injection. Otherwise, use additional contraception for 7 days.

9) A Immune, post vaccination

10) D Infected, high risk of transmission

11) C Infected, low risk of transmission

12) B Immune, past exposure to HBV

Detectable antigens/antibodies and their significance

- *sAg*: Present in acute exposure. If present longer than 6 months, represents carrier status.
- *eAg*: Indicates a high level of infectivity. Present in acute and chronic infection.
- *cAg*: Present in acute or chronic infection. Found only in liver tissue but present for life.
- *sAb (surface antibody)*: Indicates immunity following vaccination or acute infection.
- *eAb (envelope antibody)*: Indicates declining infectivity and resolving infection.
- *cAb IgM (core antibody IgM)*: Indicates recent acute infection but present for less than 6 months.
- *cAb IgG (core antibody IgG)*: Indicates past acute or chronic infection. Does not signify immunity or previous vaccination. Lifelong.

13) A The median range
If results create a normal distribution curve, the mean, median and mode are the same value. If the data are skewed, i.e. the tails of the graph are of uneven length, the mean, median and mode differ. In normally distributed data, use mean, standard deviation and 95% confidence intervals to summarize data. In non-normally distributed data, use median and range to summarize data.

14) B Cohort studies are better than other study designs for measuring the incidence of a disease in the population
A cohort study is prospective in nature. Two or more groups with different exposures are followed up to examine the outcomes. This is opposite to case-control studies where two groups with different outcomes are examined retrospectively to determine their exposures. Cohort studies might examine, for example, occupational hazards or different drug exposures. Outcome events might include side effects, disease development or complication. Cohort studies are good for examining rare exposures because you can select people to study who have had the appropriate exposure (e.g. to follow up a group of builders who have been exposed to asbestos to establish their risk of developing asbestosis compared to a group who have not been exposed to asbestos). If the **outcome** (e.g. asbestosis) is rare, it is unlikely enough cases will occur to be statistically significant.

  Case-control studies are better at looking at rare outcomes as those with the rare outcome are selected for investigation retrospectively (e.g. take a group of patients with asbestosis and a control group without asbestosis and look backwards to see who in each group has evidence of risk of asbestos exposure).

  As cohort studies occur over time, incidence of a disease can be measured. Prevalence (or point prevalence) of a disease is best looked at in cross-sectional studies as these are not carried out over time.

15) C 95%
Mean and standard deviations are a good way of summarizing a normal distribution curve. When looking at standard deviations, remember that:
- 1 standard deviation will cover approximately 68% of values
- 2 standard deviations will cover approximately 95% of values
- 3 standard deviations will cover approximately 99% of values
- 4 standard deviations will cover approximately 99.99% of values
- 1.96 standard deviations will cover exactly 95% of values.

16) B SEM=standard deviation/$\sqrt{n}$
SEM is a measure of how well the sample mean estimates the population mean. This differs from standard deviation in that SD is a measure of the spread of the values only. Standard error of the mean = standard deviation/$\sqrt{n}$ (n is the sample size).

  The SEM is smaller for larger sample sizes, so the confidence intervals are smaller for larger sample sizes. Put another way, the more patients in a study, the more precisely the study mean will approximate the actual population mean.

SEM is used to calculate confidence intervals. The interval (mean $\pm$ 1.96 SEM) is an *exact* 95% confidence interval (CI). The mean $\pm$ 2 SEM is an *approximate* 95% CI for the population mean. Remember that a 95% CI means that there is a 95% chance that the true population mean lies within the CI. This means that there is a 5% or a 1 in 20 chance that the true mean lies outside the 95% CI.

The other formulae are: standard deviation (SD) $=\sqrt{\text{variance}}$, or variance = standard deviation^2. Variance is simply another way of expressing the spread of the data.

17) A Oestrogen receptor antagonists

18) C Monoclonal antibodies against overexpression of HER2/neu oncogene

19) D Cytotoxic chemotherapeutic agents

20) A Oestrogen receptor antagonists
- Tamoxifen is the most common oestrogen receptor antagonist. Of most benefit in oestrogen receptor-positive tumours.
- Aromatase inhibitors anastrozole (Arimidex), exemestane and letrozole are used in particular in postmenopausal breast cancers.
- Trastuzumab (Herceptin) is licensed for use in early breast cancer, which overexpresses human epidermal growth factor 2 (HER2). It has been the subject of debate regarding variations in availability throughout the country. Health board variation in funding policy creates a controversial 'postcode lottery'.
- Docetaxel, paclitaxel, doxorubicin and cyclophosphamide are chemotherapeutic agents used in breast cancer. Other chemotherapeutic agents used in breast cancer are capecitabine, mitoxantrone, mitomycin and vinorelbine.
- Treatment protocols in a specialist area such as breast cancer is a moving field. Often patients become experts in their own illness and will know far more about their treatments than you do. Cancer patients are often also in phase 1 clinical trials where an agent is being used in humans for the first time. As a GP, be aware of the current available treatments as they may present in general practice. In particular, where hormonal treatment such as anastrozole or tamoxifen is to continue for 5 or more years after completion of treatment, consider whether they should be stopped during medication reviews.

21) D Catechol-O-methyltransferase inhibitors

22) F Antimuscarinic drugs

23) B Dopamine receptor (D2) agonists

24) E Monoamine oxidase-B inhibitors

All drugs work symptomatically to reduce the symptoms of tremor and rigidity that occur with idiopathic Parkinson's. The aim is to increase the level of dopamine in the brain. Dopamine cannot be given as it is emetogenic and does not cross the blood–brain barrier. Revising the different classes of drugs and their mechanism of action is worthwhile although NICE guidelines recommend that early referral for commencement of medication in secondary care is advised.

The commonly used drugs in the management of Parkinson's disease (PD) are listed below:

- *L-Dopa* is used first line in early PD, usually combined with an inhibitor of peripheral dopa-decarboxylase to minimize the dose of L-dopa required. The dose should be minimized to reduce development of motor complications (co-careldopa or co-beneldopa).
- *Dopamine receptor (D2) agonists* (bromocriptine, apomorphine, cabergoline, pergolide, pramipexole, ropinirole and rotigotine) are a possible first line treatment for early PD symptoms and in conjunction with L-dopa in later disease. Introducing dopamine agonists in the early stages of disease, before L-dopa, may postpone the development of motor complications.
- *Monoamine oxidase-B inhibitors* (selegiline, rasagiline) inhibitors may be used as a symptomatic treatment for people with early PD to delay L-dopa use, or more commonly as an adjunct to L-dopa to reduce 'end-of-dose' fluctuations.
- *Catechol-O-methyltransferase inhibitors* (entacapone and tolcapone) prevent the peripheral breakdown of L-dopa by inhibiting catechol-O-methyltransferase, allowing more L-dopa to reach the brain. It is a second line treatment licensed for use with co-beneldopa or co-careldopa in those who experience end-of-dose deterioration but who cannot be controlled on co-careldopa or co-beneldopa.
- *Antimuscarinic drugs* (benzatropine, orphenadrine, procyclidine and trihexyphenidyl/benhexol) act by reducing the effects of relative central cholinergic excess that occurs due to dopamine deficiency. These are used for drug-induced Parkinsonism more than in idiopathic PD because they are less effective than dopaminergic drugs and are associated with cognitive impairment. Benzatropine is also used as an emergency treatment for acute drug-induced dystonic reactions.
- *Beta-blockers* can be used for postural tremor in PD but do not tend to be used first line. Beta-blockers are more commonly used to treat essential tremor and tremors associated with anxiety or thyrotoxicosis.

25) A No driving licence restrictions

Age is no bar to holding a licence. A 3-year licence is issued as long as the patient at age 70 confirms with the DVLA that no medical disability is present.

26) E Disqualified from driving until treated

Persistent BP of 180/100 or greater disqualifies a Group 2 entitlement driver until BP is controlled. For Group I entitlement, continue driving unless symptomatic.

27) G Refusal or revocation

The DVLA must be notified and driving cease if cerebral metastases are present.

28) E Disqualified from driving until treated

Stop driving. Restart when symptoms are adequately controlled.

29) A No driving licence restrictions

Colour blindness is no bar to driving.

30) D 12 months off driving

A drug misuser is automatically disqualified for a minimum of 12 months. However, with close supervision on a methadone programme, he may reapply subject to annual medical review and favourable assessment.

31) A No driving licence restrictions

A single episode of fainting is no bar to driving. If loss of consciousness is a recurrent phenomenon, further investigation may be required to exclude other diagnoses. Here, the fainting is unlikely to occur at the wheel and the fainting has a clear explanation.

Driving restrictions are different depending on the type of driving licence you have. A standard car driving licence is a Group I licence. A professional licence for driving large vehicles such as HGVs is a Group 2 licence. Below is a simple summary of the restrictions for the most common scenarios GPs come across (see also www.dvla.gov.uk).

	Driving restrictions	
	Group I	Group 2
Neurological		
Faints	No restriction	No restriction
Fits	I year off	5–10 years off
Alcohol excess	6 months off	I year off
TIA/CVA		
Single	I month off	5 years
Recurrent	3 months off	Licence revoked

(*Continued*)

*Eyes**		
Requirements to drive	20 metres vision	6/9 vision
Colour blindness	No restriction	No restriction
Psychiatry		
Dementia	Doctor discretion	Licence revoked
Psychosis	3 months off	3 years off
Drug or alcohol dependence	6 months off	1 year off
Cardiovascular		
Hypertension		
Asymptomatic	No restriction	Stop if $>180/100$
Symptomatic	Stop until controlled	Stop until controlled
Arrhythmia	Stop until controlled	3 months
Pacemaker insertion	1 week off	6 weeks off
Stable angina	No restriction	6 weeks off
Unstable angina	4 weeks off	6 weeks off
Myocardial infarction	4 weeks off	6 weeks off
Coronary artery bypass graft	4 weeks off	6 weeks off
Angioplasty	1 week off	6 weeks off
Diabetes		
Diet/tablet controlled	No restrictions if well controlled and no complications	
Insulin controlled	Stop if symptomatic	Licence revoked (exceptions occasionally made depending on when licence acquired)

* Any other problem that affects vision such as visual field defects, night blindness or diplopia means driving is inappropriate until it is resolved. See also defects due to TIA/CVA.

32) D Sudden onset of hemiplegia

Hemiplegia is the most common presentation, but early recognition of the less common presentations is essential if patients are to have optimum treatment of their stroke. In acute stroke, brain imaging should be undertaken as soon as possible in all patients, at least within 24 hours. Patients should be referred as an emergency if there is:

- a known bleeding risk, e.g. patient is on warfarin or has a known bleeding tendency
- a reduced level of consciousness
- symptom progression
- headache at onset of symptoms
- a possibility of thrombolysis for thrombotic stroke.

It is imperative to refer a patient who has suffered a TIA to the rapid access TIA clinic within 1 week of the event to prevent high risk of subsequent full stroke.

33) C $<140/90$

$<140/90$ is the BP target according to NICE guidance on secondary prevention (NICE 48: 2007). A better piece of advice would be 'the lower the better' though this needs to be balanced against the possibility of side effects and cost; for example, the risk of stroke doubles between a systolic of 120 and a systolic of 140. Patients or AKT exam questions may ask about BP targets so it is helpful to be aware of them.

34) C $<140/80$

Good blood pressure control is particularly important in reducing cardiovascular risk in patients with established heart disease, diabetes or renal disease. The issue of blood pressure targets is not an easy one as there are a number of different guidelines on the subject. Below is a summary of current BP control guidelines. Refer to your local protocol for preferred targets. The Royal College however has stated that AKT exam questions will be taken from NICE guidance and BMJ Clinical Evidence.

NICE/BHS Guidelines 2006:
- Systolic/diastolic BP $>140/90$ is clinical hypertension.
- Offer drug treatment if:
  - BP $>160/100$, or
  - BP $>140/90$ if CVD risk $>20\%$, or
  - BP $>140/90$ if CVD risk $>15\%$+patient is diabetic.
  - BP target is $<140/90$ but any reduction in BP is beneficial.
  - BP target in diabetes is $<140/80$.
  - BP target in diabetes with microalbuminuria is $<135/75$.
  - Refer immediately if malignant hypertension BP $>180/110$.

Joint British Societies Guidelines:
- BP target $<140/85$ in most patients, or
- $<130/80$ if history of diabetes, stroke or heart disease, or
- $<125/75$ if diabetic with proteinuria.

RCGP CKD Guidelines:
- Treatment threshold 140/90, target 130/80 in most patients.
- Treatment threshold 130/80, target 125/75 if urine PCR >100 in CKD.

35) B $<150/80$

36) C $<145/85$

QOF targets are used for audit purposes and to calculate GMS contract payments. These are not the same as best practice targets. One of the risks of having government-set QOF targets is that GPs work towards these rather than the evidence-based targets of NICE or JSB2 guidelines, which are more beneficial to patients. QOF targets (though these may be tightened in subsequent years) are currently $<150/80$ for most patients and $<145/85$ if diabetic (QOF target for diabetes).

37) D Diclofenac

An easy mnemonic to remember the drugs that cause gout is CANT LEAP (Ciclosporin, Alcohol, Nicotinic acid, Thiazides, Loop diuretics, Ethambutol, Aspirin and Pyrazinamide). Consequently, one of the risks of anti-tuberculosis therapy is gout. Diclofenac or other NSAIDs are used in the treatment of acute gout. Colchicine can be used second line. Allopurinol is used as a prophylactic medication.

38) C Gilbert's syndrome

Gilbert's syndrome is an autosomal dominant condition producing a defect in bilirubin conjugation. It produces an increase in conjugated bilirubin which is asymptomatic ± jaundice which increases with fasting. Treatment is reassurance as it is a benign condition. Haemochromatosis is an autosomal recessive disorder of iron metabolism, leading to ferrous deposits in body tissues, including liver and pancreas, leading to 'bronze diabetes'. Wilson's disease is an autosomal recessive disorder of copper metabolism causing deposition in the liver and basal ganglia. Deposits in the cornea are known as Kayser–Fleischer rings. Budd–Chiari syndrome is caused by occlusion of the hepatic vein or inferior vena, most commonly due to thrombosis. It presents with symptoms of abdominal pain, ascites and hepatomegaly.

39) B Contemplation

40) F Decision

41) D Action

42) C Maintenance

43) E Relapse

The stages of change model was featured in the RCGP journal for Associates in Training *InnovAiT* which has some useful revision articles.

- *Pre-contemplation*: The patient is not considering change in the near future, and may not be aware of the actual or potential health consequences of continuing the harmful behaviour at this level.
- *Contemplation*: The patient may be aware of harmful consequences but is ambivalent about change.
- *Decision*: The patient has decided to change and plans to take action.
- *Action*: The patient has begun to cut down or stop their harmful behaviour, but the change has not yet become a permanent feature.
- *Maintenance*: Moderation or abstinence has been achieved on a relatively permanent basis.
- *Relapse*: Can occur at any stage. Not a failure but a learning experience to improve chances the next time round.

44) A Counselling

The 7Cs or key tasks of the Palliative Care Gold Standards Framework are as follows:

- C1 – Communication: with patient, family and between professionals.
- C2 – Coordination of care: with a named GP and district nurse for each patient.
- C3 – Control of symptoms: using symptom assessment tools and holistic approach.
- C4 – Continuity including out-of-hours: adequate anticipatory care with drugs in the home and anticipatory communication with the out-of-hours service.
- C5 – Continued learning: through audit and significant event analysis.
- C6 – Carer support: offer support as required during and after palliative care period.
- C7 – Care at the end of life: using best practice care.

45) G Meningococcal septicaemia

This is meningococcal septicaemia until proven otherwise. Treat immediately with IV/IM benzylpenicillin in the following doses: adult and child >10 yrs, 1.2 g; child 1–9 yrs, 600 mg; infant <1 yr, 300 mg. Use cefotaxime if penicillin allergic.

46) E Henoch-Schölein purpura

Henoch–Schönlein purpura presents with a painless purpuric rash over buttocks and extensor surfaces, often following a minor infection. Other features include focal segmental glomerulonephritis, joint pains and abdominal pain. It is a necrotizing capillary vasculitis and is usually self-limiting. Treatment is with bed rest and simple analgesics. Renal function should be monitored as renal failure is a complication.

47) C Gastroenteritis

Gastroenteritis is a common presentation in general practice. Many parents will be concerned about the risk of meningitis, and present for this reason. Viral gastroenteritis remains the most common cause however. Clinical assessment of hydration state is the most important aspect of the consultation. Parents should be given the opportunity to have a child reassessed if required.

48) B Bronchiolitis

Bronchiolitis is caused by respiratory syncytial virus (RSV) infection, particularly in children under 1. It can present with cough, wheeze and inability to feed due to shortness of breath. Wheeze in children under 1 is far more likely to be due to bronchiolitis (i.e. infection) rather than asthma which is allergic.

49) H Pneumonia

Left-sided basal pneumonia can present in children with left-sided abdominal pain with referred shoulder tip pain from irritation of the diaphragm via the phrenic nerve. Abdominal pain is a non-specific pain.

50) D Performers can make positive remarks

51) B Performers can make negative remarks

52) C Observers can make positive remarks

53) A Observers can make negative remarks

These are the rules to be observed when assessing any consultation performance; for example, when observing videos of consultations. This promotes a supportive, sensitive learning environment.

54) A Blue asbestos

Blue asbestos (Crocidolite), used in construction, is associated with lung cancer, mesothelioma and asbestosis. Cadmium, used in metal plating and battery manufacture, is associated with renal failure and respiratory disease. Fungal α-amylase occurs in yeasts used in bread baking. Hazardous exposures can occur in commercial bakers. It is associated with asthma. Vinyl chloride, used to produce PVC, has been associated with hepatic angiosarcoma. Wood dusts have been associated with sinonasal carcinoma.

55) B Cochlear implants

The most dangerous implants are small metallic implants where small amounts of vibration movement can cause a lot of damage (e.g. metal fragments in the eye). Cochlear implants are small and have a high capacity for vibration damage in the ear and so are contraindications to MRI. At best, the implant will fail to work following an MRI. Longstanding orthopaedic implants are not a barrier to MRI though movement may cause tingling or burning feelings. Claustrophobia is not a contraindication, though the patient may choose not to be scanned. Most tattoos can be scanned safely, but some dark blue pigments have iron particles present, which have been reported to cause burns following MRI. Piercings are not a barrier provided the patient is willing to remove them. Some heart valves can be scanned. Provide the serial number of the implant to the radiology department to assess safety. As a general rule, when referring for MRI, include any implants present on the request form. The radiographer can then assess safety.

56) C The X-ray should not be carried out after day 10 of her cycle
Lumbar spine X-rays use a higher radiation dose than other X-rays
and are subject to the '10 day rule' which states that in women of
child-bearing age, non-urgent X-ray examinations of the lumbar spine
should be restricted to the first 10 days of the menstrual cycle. The
rationale is to avoid irradiating an early pregnancy before a mother
knows she is pregnant. The 10 day rule also applies to intravenous
urograms, CTs and barium enemas. A negative pregnancy test would
not be accepted within the same cycle because before the next period is
due, it could be a false negative test. The '28 day rule' states that any
patient who has missed her period should not have any non-urgent
X-ray between the knee and the diaphragm until pregnancy has been
excluded.

57) I Female

58) J Male

59) G Deceased individual

60) D Clinically affected individual

61) C Carrier who will never manifest the disease

62) M Sex unknown

63) B Carrier for trait
Sometimes, the dark area will remain unshaded to indicate carrier status
where the trait has not yet manifest.

64) F Consultand/Index case

65) A Adopted child

66) K Monozygotic twins

67) E Consanguinity

68) H Dizygotic twins

69) N Spontaneous abortion
A shaded triangle would indicate a spontaneous abortion where the child was affected by the condition in question.

70) O Termination of pregnancy
A shaded triangle would indicate a termination of pregnancy where the child was affected by the condition in question.

71) I Parents now separated
Examiners may ask questions interpreting relationships from a pedigree diagram (family tree). Alternatively, examiners may ask candidates to identify whether the inheritance pattern of a condition is autosomal or X-linked, dominant or recessive from a pedigree chart using these symbols.

72) D Judaism
People of any faith or culture will vary in how they carry out customs. It is important to discuss relevant issues with individual patients.

73) A Left-sided conductive hearing loss
A 512 Hz tuning fork is held against the mastoid process. When the note is no longer audible, the fork is then held 1 inch (2.5 cm) from the external auditory meatus. If the sound is louder in front (air conduction), this is positive, and normal (AC > BC). If the sound is louder behind the ear, bone conduction is better than air conduction (BC > AC). This is Rinne's negative and suggests a conductive hearing loss. You can demonstrate this on yourself by plugging your ear and carrying out Rinne's test.
   The exception to this rule (a false negative) is when there is severe total ipsilateral sensorineural loss. Then, the sound will be best heard by bone conduction through the base of skull to the functioning ear on the other side. This is not the answer here, however, as the history implies a relatively mild hearing loss. To avoid false negative Rinne's, mask the contralateral ear by rubbing the tragus. If in doubt, carry out a Weber's test to differentiate. Bedside tests are not highly sensitive or specific however. Negative bedside tests should not stop you referring for audiometry with a good history.

74) A Left-sided conductive hearing loss
A 512 Hz tuning fork is held on the centre of the forehead. If the sound is localized to one side, it implies either ipsilateral conductive hearing loss or contralateral sensorineural hearing loss.

75) E There should be benefit in starting treatment early

Chlamydia is not life threatening, but there is benefit in screening. A condition does not have to affect all sections of the population. Being able to target screening towards at-risk populations is an advantage. Although screening initiatives can be carried out within an individual practice, the best screening programmes may eventually be adopted nationwide. Screening can be both opt-in or opt-out. The Wilson–Junger criteria for screening are as follows:

- an important condition
- a well understood natural history
- recognizable latent or early symptomatic stage
- test should be easily carried out and interpreted, acceptable, accurate, reliable, sensitive and specific
- acceptable treatment for cases identified by the test
- benefit in starting treatment early
- screening process should be cost effective
- screening should run as a continuous programme.

76) D Family history of atopy

Features that increase the probability of asthma include:

- more than one of the following – wheeze, cough, difficulty breathing, chest tightness, especially if frequent and recurrent
- symptoms worse at night and in the early morning
- symptoms occur in response to triggers such as exercise, pets, cold, damp
- symptoms occur in between infections
- history of atopy/family history of atopy
- wheeze heard on auscultation
- history of improvement in symptoms or lung function in response to adequate therapy.

Clinical features that lower the probability of asthma include:

- symptoms with an upper respiratory tract infection only, no interval symptoms
- isolated cough in the absence of wheeze or difficulty breathing
- history of moist cough
- prominent dizziness, light-headedness, peripheral tingling
- repeatedly normal physical examination of chest when symptomatic
- normal peak flow or spirometry when symptomatic
- no response to a trial of asthma therapy
- clinical features pointing to an alternative diagnosis.

77) D Admit to hospital for investigation

In some children, particularly the under fives, the diagnosis of asthma is not clear-cut. If there is insufficient evidence for a firm diagnosis, but no features to suggest an alternative diagnosis, there are a few appropriate options. Possible approaches are dependent on frequency and severity of symptoms and include watchful waiting with review, trial of treatment with review, spirometry and reversibility testing. Diagnostic uncertainty at this stage is not an indication for hospital referral. The diagnosis of asthma in children is a clinical one, based on recognizing a characteristic pattern of episodic symptoms in the absence of an alternative explanation.

78) A Add inhaled steroid 200 mcg/day

Below are summaries of the treatment steps in asthma. For each of the stepwise guidelines, always use the lowest step to maintain control and reassess after each step.

Management in children under 5:

Step 1 – Mild intermittent asthma: inhaled SABA as required.

Step 2 – Regular preventer therapy: add inhaled steroid 200–400 mcg/day according to severity of symptoms *or* leukotriene receptor antagonist if inhaled steroid cannot be used.

Step 3 – Initial add-on therapy: inhaled steroid *and* leukotriene receptor antagonist. In under twos, consider moving to step 4.

Step 4 – Persistent poor control: refer to respiratory paediatrician.

Management in children 5–12 years:

Step 1 – Mild intermittent asthma: inhaled SABA.

Step 2 – Regular preventer therapy: add inhaled steroid 200–400 mcg/day.

Step 3 – Initial add-on therapy: add long-acting beta-agonist (LABA). Maximize inhaled steroid. Consider leukotriene receptor antagonist or SR theophylline.

Step 4 – Persistent poor control: increase inhaled steroid up to 800 mcg/day.

Step 5 – Continuous or frequent use of oral steroids: maintain high dose inhaled steroid at 800 mcg/day. Refer to respiratory physician.

Management in adults:

Step 1 – Mild intermittent asthma: inhaled short-acting beta-2 agonist (SABA) as required.

Step 2 – Regular preventer therapy: add inhaled steroid 200–800 mcg/day, appropriate to severity of disease.

Step 3 – Initial add-on therapy: long-acting beta-agonist (LABA) and assess response. Maximize inhaled steroid. Consider leukotriene receptor antagonist or SR theophylline.

Step 4 – Persistent poor control: consider increasing steroid to 2000 mcg/day. Addition of 4th drug: leukotriene receptor antagonist, SR theophylline or beta-agonist tablet.

Step 5 – Continuous or frequent use of oral steroids: daily steroid tablet. Maintain high dose steroids. Refer for specialist care.

79) E Study e

That is the study furthest along the x-axis.

80) F Study f

That is the study furthest down the y-axis.

81) G Study g

Study g lies outwith the expected 'cone' spread of studies.

82) I 2

That is studies a, b, c, d and e, which are clear of the line of no difference.

83) P Meta-analysis shows benefit

The overall mean of all the studies appears to show clear benefit using this drug.

Funnel plots are graphs used primarily to assess bias in a meta-analysis. They plot the results of the studies published against the size of the study itself. Theoretically, the plots should form a symmetrical cone shape around the mean overall result, with smaller studies being more likely to be further away from the mean. Usually a 'cone template' is superimposed onto the graph to enable the reader to visualize the expected cone and to easily identify outlying studies. An asymmetrical funnel shape indicates either publication bias, where certain study results have not been published so as to skew the result, or systematic bias, where there is a relationship between treatment effect and the study size. The plot appears approximately symmetrical here. If it is asymmetrical, the reasons should be investigated. In the plot, the solid vertical axis represents an odds ratio of I, i.e. the line of no difference.

The dotted line represents the mean of all the studies. It is about this line that the plotted dots should be symmetrical.

This answer shows the general principles on which a funnel plot is constructed. If you are given a graph you do not recognize in the exam, the best advice is not to panic, as most answers can be worked out just using the information you have been given in the question.

84) D Where a patient is being cared for in a residential home

Consent is not automatically assumed in a care home. In particular, consent should be sought from the patient to talk to carers where they are not directly caring for the patient. Where an adverse drug reaction has occurred, it should be reported to the Medicines and Healthcare products Regulatory Agency. The most common occasion for breaching confidentiality in the interest of public health is when it is necessary to contact the DVLA to report unfitness to drive. Where a complaint has resulted in a GMC hearing, consent to use the record of the patient involved is not required.

85) D A Chinese citizen who has been in the UK for 3 weeks. He has applied for asylum

The primary decider of entitlement to free NHS treatment is that you are 'ordinarily resident' in the UK. There is no qualifying period for this, though patients who arrive in the UK are likely to be asked for evidence of the ability to legally reside in this country for more than 6 months. People who have applied for asylum immediately qualify for free NHS care, as do their children. British citizens who are leaving the country for more than 3 months are expected to surrender their NHS registration card and relinquish registration with a GP. It is not acceptable to return to the UK for short trips to take advantage of free NHS care regardless of national insurance or tax record. Foreign nationals in the UK on holiday are not entitled to free NHS care as they are not 'ordinarily resident' in the UK.

86) D Treatment for HIV diagnosed abroad but which requires ongoing treatment

Treatment for notifiable infectious diseases can be treated for free on the NHS on public health grounds. This includes tuberculosis. The exception to this is HIV where testing and counselling is free but ongoing HIV treatment will not be funded for overseas visitors to the UK. Accident and emergency treatment will be given free. Immediately necessary care in general practice can be given free on the NHS. Other free services to overseas visitors include any service from a walk-in centre of any type, and where treatment is required following an emergency psychiatric detention.

87) E Long standing bowel symptoms with alternating loose stools and constipation

The hallmarks of colorectal cancer are GI bleeding, change in bowel habit, weight loss and masses on abdominal or rectal examination.

88) B She should immediately start bone protection such as alendronate

Both male and female patients over 65 on steroids for over 3 months should be started on preventative therapy at the time of starting steroids. Scanning is not required because it would not change management. HRT should not be prescribed solely for prevention of osteoporosis.

89) B Cushing's disease

Normally dexamethasone would suppress cortisol levels to almost nothing. Failure to adequately suppress cortisol levels would suggest Cushing's disease unless there is another known cause. Alcoholism and steroid therapy can induce Cushing's *syndrome*.

90) B Betametasone nasal drops

Steroid nasal drops would be administered in the 'head down' position to shrink the polyps. Large polyps may require systemic steroids to reduce them. Once reduced, this can be maintained by using a nasal spray.

91) C Refer for intravenous Immunoglobulin

The patient is at clear risk of developing chickenpox. If the immunology showed evidence of immunity to varicella zoster, no further action would be necessary. If the patient presented with evidence of chickenpox herself, she should be referred for treatment with aciclovir and further monitoring of her pregnancy. The foetus is at risk of eye defects, hypoplasia and microcephaly.

92) A Cranial nerve I

Olfactory nerve lesions are uncommon; ear, nose and throat causes are much more common. In the absence of another explanation, olfactory nerve dysfunction can be caused by trauma, frontal lobe tumour or meningitis.

93) D Cranial nerve IV

Trochlear nerve lesions are rare in isolation but demonstrate the function of this nerve. It innervates the superior oblique muscle, which depresses and abducts the eye. May be caused by trauma to the orbit.

94) B Cranial nerve II

Multiple sclerosis with optic neuritis is the suggestion here. Optic nerve lesions could also take the form of visual field defects or acuity problems.

95) C Cranial nerve III

Lesions of the oculomotor nerve affect the medial, superior and inferior rectus and inferior oblique muscles. Damage gives a 'down and out' pupil.

96) F Cranial nerve VI

The abducens nerve innervates the lateral rectus, which abducts the eye.

97) H Cranial nerve VIII

Vestibulocochlear nerve: the vestibular nerve controls balance; the cochlear nerve controls hearing. Assess with Rinne's and Weber's tests and audiometry.

98) C Rhinovirus infection

Remember that simple presentations come up in exams too. Continue to think clearly and not overcomplicate questions. The most obvious answer is usually correct. It is not unreasonable to present to your GP when feeling unwell with an upper respiratory tract infection, though the majority of patients consult their bathroom cabinet or their pharmacist. It is appropriate to be sympathetic and give appropriate advice on this occasion.

99) D Sertraline

SSRIs should be used as a first line treatment at an age-appropriate dose. They should be tried for 6 weeks before stopping or changing medication as they can act more slowly in the elderly. Tricyclic antidepressants (TCAs) are often used for depression in the elderly but have numerous side effects – dry mouth, constipation, night sweats, drowsiness, dizziness, vivid dreams and fine tremor. Patients with cardiac arrhythmias on TCAs or with poorly controlled epilepsy should be offered SSRIs. A favourite trick is for the examiners to ask you for the second line drug treatment. So read the question carefully.

100) D Short term (up to 1 week) of low dose nitrazepam running up to his presentation is appropriate in such a stressful circumstance
Nitrazepam is a long-acting benzodiazepine. If considering prescribing benzodiazepines in this circumstance, a shorter acting drug should be used, although all carry the risk of a 'hangover' effect. Drowsiness prior to his presentation would not be an ideal outcome. Short-term prescribing for insomnia should be for no longer than 3 weeks (ideally 1 week). The other options are principles of sleep hygiene, which should be the mainstay of treatment. Other principles of sleep hygiene include avoiding daytime naps, establishing a regular bedtime routine, a warm bath and a milky drink, and avoid overstimulation with late night television. In summary, treat yourself as you would a toddler with a bedtime routine!

AKT Paper 3: Questions

1–10) *Certification in general practice*
Match the following certificates to their purpose:

A SC1
B SC2
C FW8
D SF100
E Med3
F Med4
G Med5
H Med6
I RM7
J MatB1
K MA1

1) Provided by doctor or midwife once less than 20 weeks until estimated date of delivery. Allows claim of statutory maternity pay.

2) Self-certificate to allow people in employment to claim statutory sick pay.

3) Self-certificate for self-employed or unemployed people.

4) Referral for early application of the Personal Capability Assessment.

5) Maternity claim form for prescription charge exemption.

6) Certificate for current illness lasting longer than 7 days. Must be issued within 24 hours of examination by the doctor who signs the certificate.

7) Form sent to the Department of Work and Pensions (DWP) when a vague diagnosis has been put on the certificate given to the patient. This asks the DWP to send a form requesting more precise details.

8) Form filled in by a GP prior to a patient's first application for Personal Capability Assessment.

9) Form used if a doctor has not seen a patient but is writing the certificate based on a written report from another doctor.

10) Form used for current illness where the certificate is issued >1 day since the doctor signing the certificate has examined the patient.

11) *Sex after myocardial infarction*
A 56-year-old man who had a heart attack 1 week ago comes in to discuss his new medications. He has had an uncomplicated recovery. He shifts nervously in his seat and asks when he might be able to start having sex again.
What advice do you give?

A Anytime
B 1 week post MI
C 2 weeks post MI
D 4 weeks post MI
E 3 months post MI

12) *Cervical cytology*
While reviewing incoming lab reports for your practice, you come across a cervical smear test report which states that there is 'borderline nuclear abnormality present'. The smear was taken from a 28-year-old lady. According to the request form the cervix appeared normal and the patient was suffering no symptoms. Her previous smear, taken 1 month ago, was 'inadequate'.
What further action is required?

A None
B Recall patient to surgery to discuss if there are any symptoms present
C Repeat smear immediately
D Repeat smear in 6 months
E Refer for colposcopy
F Refer for endometrial biopsy

13) *Pneumococcal vaccination*

For which one of the following conditions does the Department of Health recommend pneumococcal vaccination?

A Presence of cochlear implant
B Presence of hip replacement
C Crohn's disease
D Asthma treated with salbutamol only
E Acute pneumonia

14) *Absolute and relative risk*

A double-blind, placebo-controlled trial conducted over 5 years is testing a new drug to prevent diabetes. There were 1000 patients in the treatment arm and 1000 patients in the control arm. Over the 5-year period, 80 of the treated group developed diabetes. 100 of the group treated with placebo developed diabetes in the same period.

The correct interpretation of the data is:

A The number needed to treat to prevent one case of diabetes is 10
B The relative risk of developing diabetes is 1.25 in those treated with the new drug
C The absolute risk reduction produced by the new drug is 2%
D The relative risk reduction produced by the new drug is 2%
E The number needed to treat to prevent one case of diabetes is 8

15) *Type II statistical error*

You are reading a journal article detailing a randomized control trial of a new treatment for head lice. Your colleague thinks the study might have a type II statistical error.

Which of the following options best describes a type II statistical error?

A The statistical calculations have been incorrectly carried out
B The statistical methods selected are inappropriate
C The study shows a difference where one does not really exist
D The study shows no difference where there really is a difference
E The study question has been badly formulated

16) *Parametric and non-parametric tests*

Which of the following is an example of a parametric test?

A Student's *t*-test
B Wilcoxon rank test
C Mann–Whitney U-test
D Spearman's rank correlation
E Chi-squared test

17) *Forests plots*
Which of the following is **NOT** true in a forest or meta-analysis plot?

A Forest plots are used to summarize data from multiple different studies
B Forest plots are used to combine data when multiple studies have not reached statistical significance on their own
C The size of the squares represents the weight that the individual study contributed to the meta-analysis
D The length of the lines represents the confidence intervals
E The combined analysis is represented at the bottom by a diamond

18) *Needlestick injury*
You are working in the GP out-of-hours service and while taking a blood sample from a 24-year-old man, you have a needlestick injury.
All of the following are appropriate immediate actions to take EXCEPT:

A Wash the area thoroughly with soap and lukewarm water
B Scrub the area with chlorhexidine or betadine iodine wash
C Gently encourage bleeding
D Cover with a waterproof plaster
E Report the incident to your line manager

19) *Ottawa rules for ankle and foot X-ray*
An 18-year-old woman suffers an inverted ankle injury while on a birthday night out. She attends your surgery the following day and explains she was wearing high-heeled shoes and had been drinking. **Which of the following features would indicate that an X-ray is required to exclude a fracture?**

A Bruising over medial malleolus
B Unable to weight bear at time of injury and at time of consultation
C Patient was so intoxicated at the time she cannot remember the mechanism of injury
D Ankle swelling over lateral malleolus
E Pain remains present despite paracetamol and ibuprofen

20) *MMR vaccine*
Select TWO correct statements regarding MMR vaccination:

A Children with leukaemia are at high risk and should be offered the MMR vaccine
B The MMR vaccine contains killed viruses
C The MMR vaccine is associated with autistic enterocolitis
D The MMR vaccine is not safe in children who have had an anaphylactic reaction to eggs
E The UK recommends two doses of MMR in childhood

21) *Treatment of influenza*

During an influenza outbreak, the use of antiviral medications against influenza can potentially be used in all of the following situations EXCEPT:

A Post-exposure prophylaxis in over 65s
B Post-exposure prophylaxis in children over 1
C Prophylaxis for all residents in a care home where one resident has influenza
D Treatment of healthy individuals with influenza symptoms
E Treatment of 'at-risk' individuals with influenza symptoms

22) *Carbon monoxide poisoning*

A 30-year-old woman complains of headaches, feeling tired all the time and disoriented. She reports that she moved into a council flat in November. The flat is damp with visible mould. She also suffers from asthma and is on Dianette for contraception.

The SINGLE most appropriate management would be:

A Advise testing for carbon monoxide poisoning
B Arrange patch testing for mould sensitization
C Change Dianette to POP
D Increase inhalers since patient is allergic to mould
E Prescribe antidepressant

23) *Tinea capitis*

The SINGLE best treatment for scalp ringworm in children is:

A Clotrimazole cream
B Ketoconazole shampoo
C Oral griseofulvin
D Oral itraconazole
E Terbinafine cream

24) *Lung function testing*

A 75-year-old man attends for lung function testing following a period of shortness of breath.

In working out his predicted lung function values, which of the following DOES NOT have an influence?

A Age
B Ethnic origin
C Height
D Sex
E Weight

25–29) *Childhood rashes*
For each of the patients below select the most likely diagnosis:

A Chickenpox
B Erythema multiforme
C Erythema nodosum
D Kawasaki disease
E Hand, foot and mouth disease
F Herpes simplex
G Measles
H Molluscum contagiosum
I Scarlet fever

25) A 10-year-old boy presents with three pale umbilicated papules on his neck. He enjoys swimming at school.

26) A 3-year-old girl presents with painful mouth ulcers and red spots on her palms. She is not unwell.

27) A 15-year-old girl presents with crops of pale erythematous/violaceous macules surrounded by concentric rings on her palms. She had taken a course of penicillin.

28) A 2-year-old boy presents with high fever and a morbilliform rash that started over his forehead and cheeks and has now spread to his trunk and limbs. He has a hoarse cough and his mouth is painful and red.

29) A 7-year-old boy presents with a sore throat and a truncal rash of pink coalescent rings. He has a strawberry tongue.

30–34) *Glomerulonephropathy*
For each of the patients below select the most likely diagnosis:

A IgA nephropathy
B Minimal change glomerulonephritis
C Henoch–Schönlein purpura
D Thin membrane nephropathy
E Focal segmental glomerulosclerosis
F Mesangiocapillary glomerulonephritis
G Membranous nephropathy
H Proliferative glomerulonephritis
I Rapidly progressive glomerulonephritis

30) A 4-year-old boy presents with proteinuria, oedema and hypoalbuminuria. Renal biopsy shows fusion of podocytes on electron microscopy.

31) A 20-year-old man with HIV presents with nephrotic syndrome and hypertension. Renal biopsy shows hyalinization of glomerular capillaries and positive IF for IgM and C3.

32) A 35-year-old woman with SLE presents with renal impairment. Renal biopsy reveals thickened BM, IF positive for IgG and C3, and subepithelial deposits on electron microscopy.

33) An 80-year-old woman presents with loin pain, haematuria and fever. She was well 1 month ago. Her ESR is elevated and she has fundoscopic features of giant cell arteritis. Renal biopsy reveals a focal necrotizing glomerulonephritis with crescent formation.

34) A 10-year-old boy with sickle cell disease presents with features of nephrotic syndrome. Renal biopsy reveals large glomeruli with double basement membrane and subendothelial deposits.

35) *Antiphospholipid syndrome*
A 30-year-old woman is found to have positive antiphospholipid antibody following a second first-trimester miscarriage within 3 years.
She is at risk of all of the following EXCEPT:

A Arterial thrombosis
B Deep venous thrombosis
C Multi-infarct dementia
D Pre-eclampsia
E Placental abruption

36) *Patient-centred consultation model*
You are preparing a presentation on consultation skills. When discussing consultation technique, what does the acronym ICE stand for?

A Issues, Consequences, Examination
B Ideas, Concerns, Expectations
C Involve, Connect, Explain
D Illness, Condition, Expertise
E Initiation, Care, Enterprise

37–39) *Breast lump referral guidelines*

A woman attends your surgery concerned that she might have a breast lump.

Fill in the gaps in the algorithm regarding appropriate referral patterns.

A No lump
B Bilateral breast pain
C Dominant asymmetrical nodularity
D Unilateral breast pain
E Abscess
F Asymptomatic woman with family history of breast cancer
G Discrete lump

Guidelines for referral of patients with breast problems. (Reproduced by kind permission of NHS Cancer Screening Programmes and Cancer Research UK. Second edition revised by Austoker J, Mansel R. 2003.)

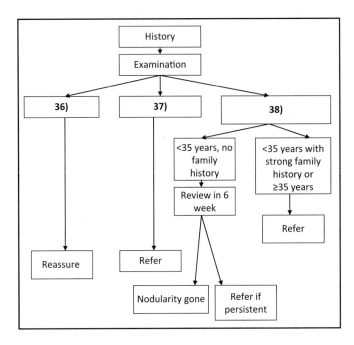

40–43) *Treatment of dermatological conditions*

For each of the patients below select the SINGLE most appropriate treatment:

A Oral flucloxacillin
B Fusidic acid cream
C Zinc and castor oil ointment
D Emollient cream
E Salicylic acid paint
F Hydrocortisone cream

40) A 4-month-old boy presents with dry skin. His mum states that his skin has been dry almost since birth and his cheeks can sometimes become red and inflamed. She has not tried any treatment.

41) A 4-month-old girl presents with nappy rash. She has a history of dry skin. Her mum uses E45 cream she bought from the chemist; however, this is not helping. On examination, the baby's buttocks are red and inflamed. The skin remains intact with no signs of bacterial or fungal infection.

42) A 1-year-old boy presents with a yellow crusting rash across the left side of his face. His mum admits to trying cream her friend gave her called fusidic acid. She tried it for a couple of days. It initially helped but the impetigo came back as soon as she stopped the cream, worse than ever. His nursery has stated that he is to be excluded until this infection has cleared.

43) A 3-year-old boy presents with a wart on his finger. It is not painful and the boy is otherwise well.

44–47) *Tropical steroids in atopic eczema*
Place the following steroid creams in order of potency as listed below:

A Betamethasone valerate 0.1% (e.g. Betnovate)
B Hydrocortisone 1%
C Clobetasol propionate 0.05% (e.g. Dermovate)
D Clobetasone butyrate 0.05% (e.g. Eumovate)

44) Mild topical steroid

45) Moderate topical steroid

46) Potent topical steroid

47) Very potent topical steroid

48) *Free prescription entitlement*
An 18-year-old woman attends your surgery. She has just started a course in childcare. She would like to know if she is entitled to free prescriptions.
Which of the following groups are NOT entitled to free prescriptions?

A A person under 18 (under 25 in Wales)
B A person under 19 and in full-time education
C A person aged 60 or over
D A person claiming income support
E A person whose partner claims income support

49) *Prescription charge exemption*
A 45-year-old man is diagnosed with type II diabetes. He asks if his diagnosis means he will no longer be required to pay a prescription charge.
Which of the following patients would be exempt from prescription charge?

A A patient suffering from chronic eczema
B A patient suffering from chronic asthma
C A patient suffering from chronic hypothyroidism
D A patient suffering from chronic hypertension
E A patient suffering from chronic obstructive pulmonary disease

50) *Qualitative research*
You wish to carry out a qualitative study to try to establish why patients continue to smoke following a quit attempt using nicotine replacement therapy.
Which of the following is NOT a qualitative research method?

A Diary methods
B Direct observation
C Focus groups
D Interview methods
E Statistical analysis

51) *Aromatherapy*
An 18-year-old woman attends your surgery asking advice regarding aromatherapy.
Which of the following is a contraindication to using aromatherapy oils?

A Second trimester of pregnancy
B Asthma
C Hay fever
D Headache
E Depression

52–57) *Herbal medicine*
For each of the following scenarios, match the complementary medicine for which there is evidence of effectiveness:

A Aloe vera
B Echinacea
C Feverfew
D Ginkgo biloba
E Horse chestnut seed extract
F Oil of Evening Primrose
G Peppermint oil
H Saw palmetto
I St John's wort
J Valerian
K Yohimbine

52) A 36-year-old woman complains of insomnia. She would like to try a herbal medicine to help her sleep.

53) A 25-year-old man suffers from occasional migraine. He would like to use migraine prophylaxis but finds that propranolol makes him very tired.

54) A 21-year-old medical student feels her mood has been low for the last 6 months. She is diagnosed with mild depression. She decides she would not like an antidepressant as she is concerned about having a history of antidepressant treatment on her medical record.

55) A 55-year-old man suffers from benign prostatic hyperplasia.

56) Psoriasis.

57) A 30-year-old woman recognizes that she gets stomach cramps and diarrhoea during stressful periods at work.

58) *Shoulder X-ray*
You are sending a patient for a shoulder X-ray.
Which of the following is the most appropriate indication for shoulder X-ray?

A Impingement
B Unstable shoulder
C Rotator cuff calcification
D Rotator cuff injury
E Muscular injury

59) *Phases of drug development*
Some of your rheumatoid arthritis patients are taking part in a double-blind, randomized control trial for a disease-modifying agent. The trial is being carried out by secondary care staff.
What type of trial is this?

A Phase 1 trial
B Phase 2 trial
C Phase 3 trial
D Phase 4 trial
E Phase 5 trial

60–64) *Automatic external defibrillator (AED) algorithm*
Complete the algorithm for automatic external defibrillation using the options below:

A 1 shock. 150–360 J biphasic or 360 J monophasic
B Continue until the victim starts to breathe normally
C Immediately resume CPR 30:2 for 2 minutes
D CPR 30:2 until AED is attached

Automatic external defibrillation (AED) algorithm

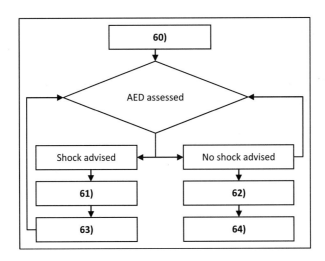

89

65) *Faith considerations*

Below is a list of considerations that may apply regarding health-care.

To which of the following World Faiths might these apply?

- Patients are likely to be vegetarians or vegans. Medications suitable for vegetarians should be offered.
- Psychosomatic techniques such as meditation may be used to ease pain. This may be preferred over oral analgesia during times of illness.
- Death should be allowed to run its natural course. Medical intervention, such as resuscitation, would interfere with this.
- A peaceful state of mind at the time of death may influence the character of rebirth.
- Some followers believe that it takes 3 days for consciousness to leave a body following death and that no disturbance or movement should take place during that time. Post mortem is normally permissible after this time.

A Buddhism
B Hinduism
C Islam
D Judaism
E Sikhism

66) *Attributable risk*

If the incidence of DVT in a high-risk population of women aged 35–45 on the combined oral contraceptive pill is 10%, and the incidence of DVT is 5% in a similar population of women who do not use the combined oral contraceptive pill, what is the value of attributable risk?

A 1%
B 2%
C 5%
D 10%
E 15%
F 25%

67) *Number needed to treat/number needed to harm*

If the incidence of DVT in a high-risk population of women aged 35–45 on the combined oral contraceptive pill is 10%, and the incidence of DVT is 5% in a similar population of women who do not use the combined oral contraceptive pill, what is the number needed to treat to prevent one event of DVT?

A 10
B 20
C 25
D 50
E 100

68–71) *Spirometry*

Interpret the following spirometry test results and match to the most likely diagnosis:

A FEV1/FVC = 66% with an FEV1 70% (obstructive)
B FEV1/FVC = 82% with an FEV1 of 60% (restrictive)
C FEV1/FVC = 40% with an FEV1 of 60% (obstructive)

68) Severe emphysema

69) Extrinsic allergic alveolitis

70) Asthma

71) Sarcoidosis

72–75) *Analgesia*

For each of the following clinical scenarios, select the MOST appropriate form of analgesia:

A Aspirin
B Diamorphine
C Diclofenac IM
D Ibuprofen
E Naratriptan
F Paracetamol
G Pizotifen
H Tramadol PO

72) A 45-year-old female presents with a 4-hour history of severe loin pain. She has no history of dysuria. She cannot get comfortable at all and has turned up at your reception desk in a state of desperation.

73) A 65-year-old man presents with severe angina. He is sweating and has taken his GTN spray. It usually takes his angina away very quickly. He has now had the pain for 15 minutes. His BP is 90/50 mmHg and his pulse is 120 bpm.

74) A 60-year-old woman with metastatic breast cancer is suffering from headache. She is asking for analgesia for this.

75) A 30-year-old woman requests analgesia for migraines. She has had these for many years but has always taken paracetamol with good effect. This is no longer helping. She is on fluoxetine.

76–81) *Antihypertensive side effects*
For each of the following side effects, match the antihypertensive drug MOST likely to be associated:

A ACE inhibitor
B Alpha-blocker
C Angiotensin receptor antagonist
D Beta-blocker
E Calcium channel antagonist
F Diuretic

76) Cold hands and feet

77) Stress incontinence

78) Headache

79) Flushing

80) Impotence

81) Dry cough

82) *Helicobacter pylori*
A 19-year-old man suffering from chronic dyspepsia tests positive for *Helicobacter pylori*.
What is the appropriate treatment?

A No treatment required
B Start proton pump inhibitor
C Proton pump inhibitor with two antibiotics
D Proton pump inhibitor with three antibiotics
E Start cimetidine

83) *Vaginal discharge*
A 21-year-old woman attends your surgery feeling unwell. She has had an offensive smelling vaginal discharge for the past week. She has a 24-hour history of fever and lower abdominal pain. Her last period was 14 days ago. She stopped taking her pill 2 months ago as she is not sexually active at present.
What is the MOST likely diagnosis?

A Retained tampon
B Bacterial vaginosis
C Pelvic inflammatory disease
D Ectopic pregnancy
E Candidal infection

84) *Polyarthritis*
A 28-year-old woman attends your surgery with a bilateral small joint polyarthritis. She is otherwise well. There have been a number of infections in her household over the past few weeks. She had a short spell of diarrhoea 3 weeks ago. Last week her daughter had a fever and bright red cheeks.
What is the MOST likely cause of the mother's illness?

A Rubella infection
B Erythrovirus B19 (formerly parvovirus B19) infection
C Rheumatoid arthritis
D Osteoarthritis
E Reiter's syndrome

85) *Bone densitometry*
When considering referring someone for bone densitometry (DEXA scanning), which of the following is NOT a major risk factor for osteoporosis?

A Premature menopause
B Cigarette smoking
C Long term steroid treatment
D Chronic liver disease
E Radiological osteopenia

86) *Immunization*
An HIV-positive patient of yours is planning to go to Africa to visit relatives during the summer. She requests advice regarding travel vaccination. Her CD4 count is 150 at present.
Which of the following vaccines would be contraindicated?

A Cholera
B Hepatitis A
C Meningococcal vaccine
D Tetanus
E Yellow fever

87) *Eczema treatment*

A 3-year-old child is diagnosed with eczema. He still wears nappies at night and his mum has found he gets terrible nappy rash when his skin flares.

Which of the following statements about this boy's skin are correct?

A The nappy rash is likely to be caused by food allergy
B His emollient should be applied first, with his steroid cream
C Cloth nappies should be used to protect his skin
D Steroid cream should be applied sparingly first, with emollients after
E Barrier creams for his nappy rash should be avoided

88) *Pulmonary tuberculosis*

A 46-year-old unemployed male patient of yours attends your surgery complaining of cough and fever. A chest X-ray is reported as having upper lobe cavitation and being strongly suspicious of tuberculosis. Urgent sputum samples are positive for tuberculosis. Your patient states that he does not want to take treatment for such an illness and that he just wanted some amoxicillin to make his cough go away. Despite repeated phone consultations and explanations, the patient still refuses to be referred to the respiratory physicians or to take treatment.

What is the MOST appropriate next step?

A No further action necessary. This is an informed decision in a competent patient.
B Give the patient 2 months to change his mind before taking further action
C Ask his wife to persuade him to take treatment
D Inform him you will be forced to contact public health if he does not willingly take treatment
E Contact the local mental health officer

89–94) *Cranial nerve lesions*

For each of the following clinical scenarios, match the affected cranial nerve:

A Cranial nerve I
B Cranial nerve II
C Cranial nerve III
D Cranial nerve IV
E Cranial nerve V
F Cranial nerve VI
G Cranial nerve VII
H Cranial nerve VIII
I Cranial nerve IX
J Cranial nerve X
K Cranial nerve XI
L Cranial nerve XII

89) A 45-year-old woman presents with a problem with her tongue. When she sticks her tongue out, it bends towards the left.

90) A 15-year-old girl presents with Bell's palsy. She has right-sided facial droop on the whole of the face. She cannot raise her eyebrows, puff out her cheeks or show her teeth.

91) A 34-year-old man presents with intractable hiccups.

92) A 70-year-old man presents with shingles. He has a painful rash across his right cheek.

93) A 60-year-old man has been diagnosed with motor neurone disease. On this occasion he presents with weakness of turning his head.

94) A 70-year-old man complains of intermittent severe pains on swallowing. He also reports his taste is not normal.

95) *Antinuclear antibody*
While reviewing your practice blood tests, you find a positive antibody result.
Which of the following is NOT associated with a positive antinuclear antibody (ANA) test?
A Drug-induced lupus
B Polymyalgia rheumatica
C Systemic lupus erythematosus
D Scleroderma
E Rheumatoid arthritis

96–100) *Autoantibodies*
Match the following disorders with the autoantibodies with which they are MOST closely associated:
A Autoimmune thyroiditis
B Goodpasture's syndrome
C Myasthenia gravis
D Rheumatoid arthritis
E Sjögren's syndrome
F Systemic lupus erythematosus
G Systemic sclerosis
H Thrombosis and recurrent miscarriage
I Wegener's granulomatosis

96) ANCA

97) Anti-Ro

98) Anti-La

99) Rheumatoid factor

100) Anti-glomerular basement membrane

AKT Paper 3: Answers

Certification questions are common. Have the differences between the Med forms clear in your head.

1) I RM7
Statutory maternity pay is paid if the woman is in employment. Women who are not entitled to maternity pay can claim maternity allowance from the DWP. Apply using form MA1. A Sure Start Maternity Grant is a one-off payment of £500, intended for people on low income. Apply using form SF100.

2) B SC2
Provides details of sickness lasting between 4 and 7 days. GPs are not obliged to issue medical certificates for periods of illness lasting less than 7 days. If a patient has been asked to provide a certificate other than a self-certificate, GPs are entitled to charge a fee.

3) A SC1
These groups are not entitled to claim statutory sick pay. Allows claim for incapacity benefit. Self-certificate for the unemployed or self-employed for periods of sickness lasting between 4 and 7 days.

4) I RM7
Sent to the DWP to request that they review the patient themselves sooner than would usually be the case. RM7 is used in difficult cases where a second opinion is required.

5) C FW8
FW8 can be filled in once a doctor or midwife has certified a pregnancy. It lasts until 12 months following the birth of the baby.

6) E Med3
Most commonly used sick line in general practice. Must be signed within a day of examining the patient.

7) H Med6
Med6 is provided when it is considered detrimental to the patient to have the accurate diagnosis on their certificate. This might, for example, be due to concerns about the employer knowing the diagnosis.

8) F Med4
Med4 is used as part of assessment by the DWP for incapacity benefit and social security.

9) G Med5

The written report cannot be more than 1 month old and the certificate cannot cover a forward period of greater than 1 month. It might be a recorded consultation with another doctor or a hospital letter for example.

10) G Med5

This is another use for the Med5. Note too that certificates are not usually issued more than once. For example, if there are two employers, one employer takes details of the certificate but does not retain it. If a certificate is lost, a replacement certificate should be clearly marked 'Duplicate'.

11) A Anytime

NICE guidelines state sex can be resumed at any time after a heart attack. Doctors can actively reassure patients and their partners that sex is no more dangerous than if they never had an MI. Sex can be resumed whenever a patient feels comfortable; most commonly around 4 weeks post MI. *Note:* Sildenafil (Viagra) is contraindicated until 6 months after MI and in patients taking nitrates.

12) D Repeat smear in 6 months

'Borderline change' indicates that it is impossible to tell if the abnormalities present are due to pre-cancerous changes, papilloma virus or inflammation. In this case a further repeat is required. If the next smear is borderline or inadequate, colposcopy is indicated. Other possible smear result codes include:

- 'Glandular neoplasia': suspicious of in-situ or invasive adenocarcinoma of cervix or endometrium. Refer for colposcopy.
- 'Severe dyskaryosis/Invasive cancer': refer for colposcopy.
- 'Severe dyskaryosis': corresponds to CIN3 (cervical intraepithelial neoplasia). Refer for colposcopy.
- 'Moderate dyskaryosis': corresponds to CIN2. Refer for colposcopy.
- 'Mild dyskaryosis': corresponds to CIN1. Repeat in 6 months. If recurrent, refer.
- 'Borderline changes': repeat in 6 months. If recurrent, refer.
- 'Inadequate': insufficient visible material for analysis. Repeat.

13) A Presence of cochlear implant

Indications for pneumococcal vaccination are as follows:

- age over 65
- asplenia or splenic dysfunction, e.g. coeliac disease (not Crohn's disease)
- chronic respiratory, heart, renal or liver disease (not acute)
- tablet- or insulin-treated diabetes
- immune deficiency due to disease, e.g. HIV, or medication such as steroids

- cochlear implant
- conditions where CSF leakage may occur
- children under 5 with a history of invasive pneumococcal disease.
Note: Asthma is only an indication if treated with frequent or continuous systemic steroids.

14) C The absolute risk reduction produced by the new drug is 2%
   - CER (control event rate) = 10%
   - EER (experimental event rate) = 8%
   - ARR (absolute risk reduction (or increase)) = CER − EER = 2%
   - RRR (relative risk reduction (or increase)) = (CER − EER)/ CER = 0.2 or 20%.
   - NNT (number needed to treat/number needed to harm) = 1/ARR = 50.

15) D The study shows no difference where there really is a difference
   The null hypothesis is always that there is no difference between groups under study. A type I error occurs when the null hypothesis is falsely rejected or, to put it another way, to state there is a significant difference between the items studied when the observation actually occurred by chance or by bad study design. A type II error occurs when the null hypothesis is falsely accepted, i.e. to see no difference between the study and control groups where there is in fact a difference.

16) A Student's *t*-test
   Parametric tests assume that data are normally distributed. If your study data are not normally distributed, a non-parametric test should be used. Examples of parametric tests are:
   - *Student's t-test*: a test of the null hypothesis comparing the means of two samples.
   - *Pearson's correlation coefficient*: a measure of the strength of a relationship between two variables. Think of correlation as 'co-relation' − a measure of how two variables are related, usually the relationship between an exposure and an outcome.
   For non-normally distributed data, non-parametric tests are used. These are usually based on ranking data. Non-parametric tests are:
   - *Wilcoxon signed rank test*: an alternative to the paired student's *t*-test comparing two related sample means or repeated measurements on a single sample.
   - *Mann-Whitney U-test*: a test used to compare data from two independent groups of samples. It identifies whether the two samples are from identical or non-identical populations.
   - *Kendall tau rank correlation coefficient*: a test measuring the degree of correspondence between two rankings and assessing the significance of their correspondence. In other words, it measures the strength of association between two groups.
   - *Spearman's rank correlation*: another non-parametric test that measures the strength of a relationship between two variables.
   - *Chi-squared test*: used to compare proportions between two groups of non-continuous data.

Remember that when using any statistical test, finding that an exposure and an outcome are *correlated* does not necessarily mean *causation*.

The nMRCGP curriculum states that candidates are to be aware of various statistical tests but are not required to know how to carry these out.

17) B Forest plots are used to combine data when multiple studies have not reached statistical significance on their own

Forest plots are used in meta-analyses to summarize data from multiple studies. They comprise a central square with lengths of horizontal lines emerging from them. The size of the squares represents the weight that the individual study contributed to the meta-analysis. The length of the lines represents the confidence intervals, though not always 95% confidence intervals. In general, the larger the study, the narrower the confidence interval and the larger the square. It then follows that the studies with the largest squares will tend to have the smallest confidence intervals. The overall estimate from the meta-analysis and its confidence interval are put at the bottom, represented as a diamond. The centre of the diamond represents the pooled point estimate, and its horizontal tips represent the confidence interval. Significance is achieved at the set level if the diamond is clear of the line of no effect.

18) B Scrub the area with chlorhexidine or betadine iodine wash
Immediate action to be taken in the event of a needlestick injury or other contaminating incident involving body fluids is as follows:
- wash the site liberally with soap and water. Do not scrub
- irrigate mucous membranes or conjunctivae with large quantities of water
- bleeding must be gently encouraged for puncture wounds
- do not suck the site
- report the incident immediately to your line manager and assess the risk involved
- contact occupational health.

Accident and Emergency Department attendance is not usually necessary unless the wound needs stitched or HIV prophylaxis is required.

19) B Unable to weight bear at time of injury and at time of consultation
Ottawa rules for ankle injuries
Refer for ankle X-ray if there is pain in the malleolar area **and** any one of the following:
- bone tenderness at the posterior tip of the lateral malleolus
- bone tenderness at the posterior tip of the medial malleolus
- patient is unable to weight bear at the time of the injury and when seen.

Ottawa rules for foot injuries
Refer for foot X-ray if there is pain in the midfoot **and** any one of the following:
- bone tenderness at the 5th metatarsal base
- bone tenderness at the navicular bone

- patient is unable to weight bear at the time of the injury and when seen.

Otherwise, diagnose a sprain or other injury (possibly can't definitely say that is a sprain?).

20) A Children with leukaemia are at high risk and should be offered the MMR vaccine

E The UK recommends two doses of MMR in childhood

MMR contains live, attenuated viruses. It does not contain any egg. Contraindications to MMR include:

- children with severe immunosuppression
- children who have had another live vaccine by injection within 4 weeks
- children who have had an anaphylactic reaction to exipients such as gelatin and neomycin.

If given to women, pregnancy should be avoided for the next month. No other chronic disease should be a barrier to immunization.

21) D Treatment of healthy individuals with influenza symptoms

Symptomatic treatment is still the mainstay of treatment in influenza. Recommend regular paracetamol, fluids and rest. Antivirals can be used for prophylaxis to reduce the duration of symptoms and reduce frequency of complications. There are three licensed medications for the prophylaxis and treatment in influenza (oseltamivir, zanamivir and amantadine). Each drug has slightly different indications in influenza A, B and C. The guidelines can be summarized as follows:

- treatment is recommended in 'at-risk' individuals as soon as possible after the onset of symptoms but can be started up to 48 hours
- treatment is not recommended in otherwise healthy individuals with symptoms of influenza
- Post-exposure prophylaxis is indicated in 'at-risk' individuals
- post-exposure prophylaxis is not indicated in otherwise healthy individuals
- seasonal prophylaxis is not recommended in any individual
- as of February 2006, oseltamivir is licensed for use in children over 1
- at-risk categories include patients over the age of 65, patients with chronic respiratory disease, diabetes, significant CV disease (excluding hypertension), chronic renal disease, and those with immuno-suppression

22) A Advise testing for carbon monoxide poisoning

The flat may not have central heating and if the walls are mouldy then concern arises as to whether there is a gas leak from poor gas maintenance. Carbon monoxide poisoning increases during winter and the risk of dying is greater in the 2 million households that rely on solid fuel. Carbon monoxide binds preferentially to haemoglobin rather than oxygen, leading to consequent tissue anoxia. Toxicity can present subtly over weeks causing headaches and mild shortness of breath on exertion. Severe toxicity results in confusion, coma and fits. Treatment is by high flow oxygen and hyperbaric oxygen where available.

23) C Oral griseofulvin

Scalp ringworm (tinea capitis) is a common childhood infection. The *BNF for Children* suggests systemic treatment first line as topical treatment is unlikely to be effective. Effective treatment is essential as scalp ringworm can cause permanent scarring and hair loss. Only oral griseofulvin is licensed in the UK to treat tinea capitis in children. Antifungal creams do not penetrate the hair shaft. Antifungal shampoos that contain selenium sulphide or povidone can be used in early infection and to treat family members to reduce the risk of infection.

24) E Weight

For FEV1 and FVC measurements, reduce values by 7% for Asians and 13% for African–Caribbeans. Men have greater lung function than women. Height affords better lung function. Lung function increases in puberty, then from around the mid-30s, gradually deteriorates with age. Weight has no influence on lung function testing.

25) H Molluscum contagiosum

Molluscum contagiosum comprises painless, pale, pearly pink papules with a central umbilicus. Spread by direct skin contact. They can be squeezed to remove the central core, which can speed immune response and resolution but can cause scarring. A self-limiting disease.

26) E Hand, foot and mouth disease

Hand, foot and mouth disease is caused by Coxsackie A virus. The lesions form on the feet, palms, buccal mucosa and sometimes buttocks. The lesions are tender clear vesicles with a surrounding erythema which burst and ulcerate. A self-limiting condition, treat symptomatically with Bonjela gel. It is sometimes wise to reassure parents that this is unrelated to foot and mouth disease in cattle.

27) B Erythema multiforme

Erythema multiforme presents as painless target lesions on the hands and feet. 50% are idiopathic. Infective causes are streptococcus, HSV, Hep B and mycoplasma. Drug causes include penicillin, sulphonamides and barbiturates.

28) G Measles

Measles presents initially with non-specific symptoms – fever, conjunctivitis, cough and coryza. Koplik's spots on the buccal mucosa and the classic rash appear later. Ask about vaccination. If suspected, contact public health for local advice on confirmation. Treatment is symptomatic only.

29) I Scarlet fever

Scarlet fever is caused by Group A strep and has an incubation period of 2–4 days. Presents with fever, headache, tonsillitis, a fine punctuate rash, scarlet facial flushing and a 'strawberry' tongue. It is treated with penicillin V and is an important infection because of the risk of rheumatic fever and acute glomerulonephritis.

30) B Minimal change glomerulonephritis
This is a case of nephrotic syndrome – proteinuria, oedema and hypoalbuminuria. Minimal change glomerulonephritis is most common in children. Corticosteroids induce remission in >90% of children.

31) E Focal segmental glomerulosclerosis
There is a poor response to corticosteroids (10–30%) and there is a high risk of chronic renal failure. Cyclophosphamide or ciclosporin may be used.

32) G Membranous nephropathy
Other associations include malignancy, drugs, autoimmune conditions and infections. Treatment involves corticosteroids and chlorambucil (Ponticelli regimen). It has a high risk of progression to chronic renal failure.

33) I Rapidly progressive glomerulonephritis
Treatment involves high-dose corticosteroids, cyclophosphamide 5 plasma exchange or renal transplant. Prognosis is poor if the initial serum creatinine level is >600 μmol/L.

34) F Mesangiocapillary glomerulonephritis
There is no treatment and half will progress to end-stage renal failure. Take home messages include consideration of renal disease in presentations of hypertension, peripheral oedema, fever and joint pain. Urinalysis will show proteinuria and/or haematuria. Other diagnoses to consider are adult polycystic kidney disease, renal vein thrombosis and renal artery stenosis.

35) E Placental abruption
Antiphospholipid syndrome occurs with SLE, or independently, and requires close supervision during pregnancy due to increased clotting tendency. Mothers are commenced on aspirin and may require subcutaneous heparin or warfarin. The baby is at risk of placental insufficiency, IUGR and fetal death. Other associations include migraine, myelitis, stroke and myocardial infarction.

36) B Ideas, Conserns, Expectations
Patients' health beliefs can be broken down into ideas, concerns and expectations. These affect patients' consulting behaviour. Taking these into consideration will increase the likelihood of treatment compliance and will improve patient satisfaction with the consultation.

37) A No lump

38) G Discrete lump

39) C Dominant asymmetrical nodularity
Although the other options could be filled in appropriately, this algorithm refers to breast lump referral guidelines and should be familiar. Prior to the AKT, familiarize yourself with local protocol algorithms as these will always be based on national guidelines.

40) D Emollient cream
The diagnosis here is likely atopic eczema. In the first instance, advice on skincare is all that is required. Steroid creams should be reserved for flares and used as sparingly as possible.

41) C Zinc and castor oil ointment
Nappy rash is common and most parents will have tried various over-the-counter nappy creams before presenting to their GP. A barrier cream such as zinc and castor oil cream is all that is required. Signs of fungal or bacterial infection should prompt treatment with clotrimazole or fusidic acid cream respectively, with or without additional steroid cream.

42) A Oral flucloxacillin
Impetigo, although a benign condition, spreads rapidly among children in schools and nurseries. It is common to have a policy of exclusion. Small areas of impetigo can be treated with topical fusidic acid, but resistance occurs quickly. Larger areas are best treated with systemic flucloxacillin. It is wise to warn parents that flucloxacillin is quite unpalatable. A dose quickly followed by juice can make it easier for children to take.

43) E Salicyclic acid paint
Warts are a common benign condition. No treatment is a valid option, with reassurance that it will settle with time. Salicylic acid gel applied to the wart surface only will wear down the hyperkeratosis. The wart should then be worked on with a pumice stone. Liquid nitrogen can be used but is painful. Verrucas are simply plantar warts and should be treated in the same way.

44) B Hydrocortisone 1%

45) D Clobetasone butyate 0.05% (e.g. Eumovate)

46) A Betamethasone valerate 0.1% (e.g. Betnovate)

47) C Clobetasol propionate 0.05% (e.g. Dermovate)
Patients tend to refer to steroid creams by their trade names. AKT questions are likely to refer to generic names only. Patients who have had eczema for a long time will be familiar with the relative strengths of different creams. It is wise to be familiar with these. The most commonly prescribed creams of each strength are listed below, along with a brand name. The top cream on each list is the most commonly prescribed.
Steroid cream potencies
The top creams on each list are the most commonly prescribed.

Mild

- hydrocortisone 0.1–2.5%
- there are many branded variants with additional active ingredients such as urea, clotrimazole or fusidic acid

Moderate

- betamethasone valerate 0.025% (1 in 4 dilution of Betnovate cream–betamethasone 0.1%)
- alclometasone dipropionate 0.05% (e.g. Modrasone)
- clobetasone butyrate 0.05% (e.g. Eumovate)
- fludroxycortide 0.0125% (e.g. Haelan)
- fluocortolone caproate 0.25% (e.g. Ultralanum Plain).

Potent

- betamethasone valerate 0.1% (e.g. Betnovate)
- betamethasone dipropionate 0.05% (e.g. Diprosone)
- hydrocortisone butyrate 0.1% (e.g. Locoid)
- Fluocinolone acetonide 0.025% (e.g. Synalar)
- fluocinonide 0.05% (e.g. Metosyn)
- fluticasone propionate (e.g. Cutivate)
- mometasone furoate (e.g. Elocon).

Very potent

- clobetasol propionate 0.05% (e.g. Dermovate)
- diflucortolone valerate 0.1–0.3% (e.g. Nerisone)

According to NICE guidance, choice of steroid cream should be guided by the severity of the eczema as summarized below:
- mild eczema should be treated with a mild potency steroid cream
- moderately severe eczema should be treated with a moderately potent steroid cream
- severe eczema should be treated with a potent steroid cream
- eczema should be treated with the least potent steroid cream required to control symptoms. It should be applied to affected areas only

- steroid creams should be applied thinly to affected areas only in 'fingertip units'
- a fingertip unit (around 500 mg) is the cream squeezed from the tip of the adult index finger to the first crease. This should be adequate to cover an area that is twice that of the flat adult palm.

Emollients remain the mainstay of treatment in atopic eczema.

48) A A person under 18 (under 25 in Wales)
The true statement would be 'A person under 16 (under 25 in Wales)'.
The following are entitled to free prescriptions:

- if you are under 16 (under 25 in Wales)
- if you are under 19 and in full-time education
- if you are aged 60 or over
- if you (or your partner) gets Income Support, Income-based Jobseeker's Allowance or Pension Credit Guarantee Credit
- if you have an NHS tax credit exemption certificate
- some war pensioners – if treatment is connected with the pensionable disability
- if you have a prescription exemption certificate (see below)
- if you are pregnant or have had a child in the past year.

49) C A patient suffering from chronic hypothyroidism
The following conditions confer exemption from prescription charge:

- a permanent fistula requiring dressing
- forms of hypoadrenalism such as Addison's disease
- diabetes insipidus and other forms of hypopituitarism
- diabetes mellitus except where treatment is by diet alone
- hypoparathyroidism
- myasthenia gravis
- myxoedema (underactive thyroid) or other conditions where supplemental thyroid hormone is necessary
- epilepsy requiring regular anti-epilepsy medication
- permanent physical disability with reduced mobility.

50) E Statistical analysis
Qualitative research is carried out to answer questions which cannot be easily answered using quantitative research, i.e. where things cannot be numerically measured. In particular, qualitative research is concerned with opinions, attitudes and beliefs. Statistical analysis must involve numerical measurements, which do not occur in qualitative research.

- diary methods – where daily written accounts are analysed
- direct observation – where an external observer records events
- focus groups – where a subject is discussed and the transcription analysed
- interview methods – where an individual is interviewed and the exchange analysed.

51) A Second trimester of pregnancy

It is common for patients to ask our advice about over-the-counter remedies, especially if a product has been in the news. There is very little evidence for the effectiveness of aromatherapy oils but there are some known contraindications:

- pregnancy – avoid basil, cedarwood, clary sage, juniper berry, marjoram, myrrh and sage
- epilepsy – avoid fennel, sage and rosemary
- hypertension – avoid rosemary, sage, thyme and stimulating spice oils
- citrus oils and bergamot should be avoided prior to sun exposure

52) J Valerian

Valerian root is sold over the counter in 'daytime' preparations for anxiety and 'nighttime' preparations for insomnia.

53) C Feverfew

Feverfew has been used for headaches but it has stronger evidence for migraine prophylaxis and reduction of migraine severity.

54) I St John's wort

There is strong evidence for the use of St John's wort (*Hypericum perforatum*) as a first line antidepressant. In Germany, it is licensed for use in anxiety, depression and insomnia. *Note*: It should not be used in conjunction with prescription antidepressants. There are also concerns that it is a liver enzyme inducer and can therefore interact with medications metabolized in the liver. Patients are often concerned about having a record of mental illness on their medical record, and so may seek treatment via an over-the-counter solution.

55) H Saw palmetto

Finasteride is considered to be best used in men with larger prostate volumes. Finasteride should therefore be used first line in men with larger prostate volume. The evidence for saw palmetto is better for those with milder disease. It is thought to have a better side effect profile than finasteride.

56) A Aloe vera

There is some evidence from randomized, double-blind trials to show that aloe vera is effective for psoriasis and genital herpes; however, there is no high-quality evidence for effectiveness of aloe vera for wound healing, radiation-induced skin injury, hyperlipidaemia or diabetes mellitus.

57) G Peppermint oil

There is some evidence for the use of peppermint oil to reduce the symptoms of irritable bowel syndrome; however, it is associated with the following side effects: heartburn, perianal burning, blurred vision, nausea and vomiting.

The problem with herbal medicines is that the trials are all very small and side effects unmonitored. Kava is a herbal medicine with evidence of effectiveness in anxiety. Products sold in the UK were removed from sale in 2002 due to reports of severe liver toxicity.

Herbal supplements with evidence of efficacy

- echinacea: prevention and treatment of the common cold
- ginkgo biloba: may help tinnitus, intermittent claudication and improve cerebral blood flow
- chinese herbal medicine: evidence for childhood eczema and IBS. Has been associated with renal dysfunction
- oil of Evening Primrose: rheumatoid arthritis
- horse chestnut seed extract: chronic venous insufficiency
- yohimbine: erectile dysfunction.

58) C Rotator cuff calcification

X-ray can be used to show calcific tendonitis deposits, which will be radio-opaque. X-rays can also be used in episodes of trauma to diagnose fractures or dislocations. X-rays however are unhelpful for most other rotator cuff problems, impingement, instability or muscular injuries. Impingement can be diagnosed clinically. Ultrasound and MRI are better at functionally imaging the shoulder, though these are not universally available.

59) A Phase I trial

- Phase 1 – Animal model trials. First trial of a compound in human volunteers. Primarily testing safety in humans rather than effectiveness
- Phase 2 – Therapeutic trials in patients. Now testing beneficial effects rather than just safety
- Phase 3 trials – Randomized controlled trials
- Phase 4 trials – Post marketing surveillance.

Because of the nature of some drugs (e.g. chemotherapeutic agents), phase I trials are carried out in a patient population rather than healthy human volunteers because it would be unethical to give a cytotoxic agent to healthy volunteers.

60) D CPR 30:2 until AED is attached

61) A 1 shock. 150–360 J biphasic or 360 J monophasic

62) C Immediately resume CPR 30:2 for 2 minutes

63) C Immediately resume CPR 30:2 for 2 minutes

64) B Continue until the victim starts to breathe normally
Manual defibrillators tend to be used in hospital although automatic external defibrillators are being introduced into hospital wards to widen the range of staff who can defibrillate patients. Staff more comfortable using a manual system can easily override an automatic device to use it manually. Automatic external defibrillators are more likely to be used in the community, not only in general practice but also in community and shopping centres to allow members of the public to quickly respond in an arrest. Resuscitation algorithms lend themselves to algorithm completion AKT questions.

65) A Buddhism
People of any faith or culture will vary in how they carry out customs. It is important to discuss relevant issues with individual patients.

66) C 5%
Attributable risk is the incidence in the exposed population minus the incidence in the non-exposed population.

67) B 20
The number needed to harm (NNH) is the inverse of the attributable risk (AR). The attributable risk is the incidence in the exposed population minus the incidence in the non-exposed population. If the analysis was looking at a treatment, the equivalent calculation would look at the number needed to treat (NNT).
- NNH or NNT = 1/AR
- AR = 10% −5% = 5%
- NNT or NNH = 1/(5%) = 100/5 = 20

68) C FEV1/FVC = 40% with an FEV1 of 60% (obstructive)
Emphysema is an obstructive disease. In obstructive disease, the FEV1/FVC ratio is <70% with an FEV1 of <80% predicted. In restrictive disease, the FEV1/FVC ratio is >70% with an FEV1 of <80% predicted. Normally, the FEV1 should be >80% predicted with an FEV1/FVC ratio between 70% and 80%.

69) B FEV1/FVC = 82% with an FEV1 of 60% (restrictive)
Extrinsic allergic alveolitis is a restrictive lung disease.

70) A FEV1/FVC = 66% with an FEV1 of 70% (obstructive)
Asthma is an obstructive lung disease.

71) B FEVI/FVC=82% with an FEVI of 60% (restrictive)
Sarcoidosis is a restrictive lung disease.

	Obstructive	Restrictive	Mixed
FEVI	↓	↓ or −	↓
FVC	↓ or −	↓	↓
FEVI/FVC	↓	↑ or −	↓

The FEVI (forced expiratory volume in I second) is the volume of
air expelled in the first second of maximal forced expiration from full inspiration. Anything over 80% predicted is considered normal. Both
restrictive and obstructive lung diseases will reduce FEVI.

The FVC (forced vital capacity) is the maximum volume expired after a
single maximal inspiration, normally between 3 and 6 litres depending
on height, gender and age. Normal is considered to be >80% predicted.
The FVC is reduced in both obstructive and restrictive respiratory
disease.

The FEVI/FVC ratio is the ratio of the forced expiratory volume in I
second to the forced vital capacity of the lungs. Normal is >70%
predicted. Obstructive lung diseases have an FEVI/FVC <70%. Restrictive
lung diseases have a normal or high FEVI/FVC ratio. In patients
with obstructive lung disease, the FEVI is disproportionately reduced as
compared to the FVC, resulting in a low FEVI/FVC ratio. In patients
with restrictive pulmonary disease, the FEVI and FVC fall proportionately,
resulting in normal values for FEVI/FVC.

Restrictive lung disease (due to reduced compliance)

- asbestosis
- radiation fibrosis
- drug-induced interstitial fibrosis
- idiopathic pulmonary fibrosis
- sarcoidosis
- extrinsic allergic alveolitis.

Obstructive lung disease (due to airway narrowing)

- cOPD – both emphysema and chronic bronchitic elements
- asthma
- cystic fibrosis
- bronchiectasis
- bronchiolitis
- allergic aspergillosis.

72) C Diclofenac IM
Diclofenac IM or PR is the best analgesic for renal colic. An alternative
would be IM pethidine.

73) B Diamorphine

Administer diamorphine, but also give aspirin while awaiting the ambulance. Morphine is an acceptable alternative but diamorphine is faster acting.

74) H Triamadol PO

If dexamethasone were an option here, this might be an alternative, though it would have to be clear that brain metastases were present. Other than that, moderate potency opiates are appropriate.

75) E Naratriptan

Simple analgesia should be the first line treatment for migraine. At first sign, take a full dose of aspirin, paracetamol or ibuprofen. Soluble tablets are acceptable in this situation due to the need for rapid action. Antiemetics are a useful addition. Triptans can be used as a second line treatment. Clear instructions should be given regarding their use. The tablet should be taken as soon as possible after symptoms start but not in the aura phase. If the headache recurs within 24 hours a second dose can be taken. If a first dose is not successful, reconsider the diagnosis. If the diagnosis is clear, but oral triptans are ineffective, consider nasal triptans. Beta-blockers, sodium valproate, pizotifen can be considered as prophylaxis. Start pizotifen at a low dose to avoid drowsiness. Amitriptyline can be helpful as prophylaxis, especially if tension headaches also feature.

76) D Beta-blocker

Beta-blockers are contraindicated in asthma and their main side effects are gastrointestinal disturbances, bradycardia, hypotension, headache, peripheral vasoconstriction and fatigue.

77) B Alpha-blocker

Alpha-blockers are used in hypertension and to treat prostatic hyperplasia. Their main side effects are postural hypotension, dizziness, vertigo, fatigue and asthenia. Stress incontinence is a rare side effect.

78) E Calcium channel antagonist

The main side effects of calcium channel blockers are abdominal pain, nausea, palpitations, flushing, oedema and headache. Rate-limiting calcium antagonists can cause bradycardia and sinoatrial or AV block.

79) E Calcium channel antagonist

The main side effects of calcium channel blockers are abdominal pain, nausea, palpitations, flushing, oedema and headache. Rate-limiting calcium antagonists can cause bradycardia and sinoatrial or AV block.

80) F Diuretic

Although also associated with angiotensin receptor antagonists, this side effect is more common in diuretic users. The other primary side effects patients complain of are frequency and nocturia.

81) A ACE inhibitor

It is common to have to switch patients from an ACE inhibitor to an angiotensin receptor antagonist because of dry cough. The side effect is reversible on switching therapy.

This is a difficult question. Whereas candidates are not expected to memorize the *BNF*, being aware of side effects of commonly used medications demonstrates an experience of prescribing in general practice. As you learn about medications commonly used in general practice, take note of side effects you come across, especially where side effects are characteristic of a particular drug.

82) C Proton pump inhibitor with two antibiotics

Eradication of *Helicobacter pylori* reduces recurrence of gastric and duodenal ulcers. One week of acid suppression and two antibiotics is the necessary treatment. The most common combination therapy is a proton pump inhibitor, clarithromycin and either metronidazole or amoxicillin. Most microbiology departments rotate their locally recommended treatment regimens to prevent resistance.

83) A Retained tampon

Ectopic pregnancy and pelvic inflammatory disease should be considered but given the history, retained tampon is the most likely diagnosis. This should be easily identified on pelvic examination. This lady is at risk of toxic shock syndrome if untreated.

84) B Erythrovirus B19 (formerly parvovirus B19) injection

The child has had 'slapped cheek syndrome', which is caused by erythrovirus B19 (formerly parvovirus B19). In children, the illness is generally mild. It tends to present more severely in adults with the triad of fever, rash and arthritis. A pregnant woman with a known contact with erythrovirus should have her immune status checked. At <20 weeks, there is an increased miscarriage rate or anaemia in the foetus. If infection is suspected, refer for early transfusion.

85) B Cigarette smoking

Major risk factors for osteoporosis include:
- untreated hypogonadism: premature menopause, secondary amenorrhoea and primary hypogonadism (in women or men)
- long-term steroid therapy (7.5 mg/day for > 6 months)
- diseases increasing the risk of osteoporosis – gastrointestinal disease, chronic liver disease, hyperparathyroidism, hyperthyroidism

- radiological osteopenia.

Other risk factors not included as 'major' risk factors in the RCP guidelines are:

- low bodyweight
- height loss
- family history
- cigarette smoking.

DEXA scanning should be carried out on people who have had a previous fragility fracture if they have major risk factors. Most local referral centres will not accept minor risk factors as a reason for referral as services are limited in most areas.

86) E Yellow fever

Yellow fever is a live attenuated vaccine and is contraindicated in immunocompromised individuals. Meningococcal A/C is a polysaccharide vaccine; cholera and hepatitis A are inactivated vaccines; tetanus is a toxoid. Polio and typhoid are usually inactivated vaccines in the UK, but are available as live vaccines. Yellow fever vaccine certification may be required to enter certain countries. HIV per se is no barrier to vaccination if disease is under control.

87) D Steroid cream should be applied sparingly first, with emollients after

Applying steroid creams as a second layer significantly affects the dilution and therefore the effectiveness of the cream. Eczema at this age is not likely to be specifically linked to allergy. His nappy rash is due to the increased fragility of the skin. Cloth nappies tend not to be so good at avoiding this. Modern disposable nappies are very good at absorbing moisture.

88) D Inform him you will be forced to contact public health if he does not willingly undertake treatment

In a circumstance like this, public health becomes the priority. The patient is not suspected of having a mental health problem, and appears to be mentally competent, so cannot be detained under the Mental Health Act. He does have open pulmonary tuberculosis, however, and poses a public health risk. The local public health team should be contacted. The team will try also to persuade the patient to have treatment voluntarily. If unsuccessful, they can apply through the courts to have the patient detained for treatment under the Public Health Act. In practice, however, this rarely becomes necessary.

89) I Cranial nerve XII

The hypoglossal nerve provides innervation to the muscles of the tongue. Also used in speech articulation in the sounds 'la' and 'ta'. On tongue protrusion, the tongue deviates to the side of the lesion. Can be caused by trauma or cranial tumours.

90) G Cranial nerve VII

An upper motor neurone lesion would spare the forehead. The facial nerve supplies the muscles of facial expression and the anterior two-thirds of the tongue.

91) J Cranial nerve X

The vagus nerve supplies the muscles of swallowing and parasympathetic supply to the thorax and abdomen. It also regulates most of voice control and the gag reflex. It is the parasympathetic supply to the diaphragm that causes hiccups.

92) E Cranial nerve V

This is shingles with trigeminal neuralgia. The trigeminal nerve has motor and sensory components. Its motor function is to open the mouth. Damage means the open jaw deviates to the side of the lesion. Its sensory function covers facial sensation and corneal reflex. Shingles can affect any of the three branches of the trigeminal nerve.

93) K Cranial nerve XI

The accessory nerve controls the muscles of the neck, in particular the trapezius and sternomastoid muscles. Damage causes weakness of shoulder shrugging and weakness of head movement.

94) I Cranial nerve IX

The glossopharyngeal nerve supplies taste and sensation to the posterior two-thirds of the tongue. It supplies the parotid salivary gland. This gentleman has glossopharyngeal neuralgia.

95) B Polymyalgia rheumatica

Antinuclear antibodies (ANAs) are directed against a variety of nuclear antigens. They are identified by direct immunofluorescence. Different patterns of immunofluorescence staining can indicate different disorders but none is specific enough to be diagnostic. Interpret these tests with caution. ANAs are found in:
- drug-induced lupus
- SLE
- scleroderma
- Sjögren's syndrome
- mixed connective tissue disease
- polymyositis.

96) I Wegener's granulomatosis

97) E Sjögren's syndrome

98) E Sjögren's syndrome

99) D Rheumatoid arthritis

100) B Goodpasture's syndrome
Autoantibodies and their associations are common exam multiple choice questions.

Antibodies and their associations

- acetylcholine receptor antibody – myasthenia gravis
- aNCA/cANCA – Wegener's granulomatosis and microscopic polyangiitis (40% of cases)
- aNCA/pANCA – microscopic polyangiitis (60%)
- anti-thyroglobulin – autoimmune thyroiditis
- antiphospholipid (also detected as lupus anticoagulant and anticardiolipin antibodies) – associated with arterial and venous thrombosis and recurrent miscarriage
- anti-glomerular basement membrane – Goodpasture's syndrome
- anti-Ro – Sjögren's syndrome, congenital heart block, ANA-sensitive SLE
- anti-La – primary Sjögren's syndrome
- anti-Sm – SLE. Only in 20% of cases but it suggests a high risk of renal lupus
- anti-RNP – mixed connective tissue disease, SLE
- anti-Jo1 – polymyositis
- anti-Scl70 – systemic sclerosis
- anti-centromere – CREST syndrome
- dsDNA – SLE
- anti-reticulin – coeliac disease
- anti-gastric parietal cell – pernicious anaemia
- rheumatoid factor – rheumatoid arthritis and polyarteritis.

(Anti-Ro, anti-La, anti-Sm, anti-RNP, anti-Jo1, anti-Scl70 and anti-centromere antibodies are all specific antinuclear antibodies and so are usually associated with positive ANA. Remember CREST syndrome comprises **C**alcinosis, **R**aynaud's, o**E**sophageal dysmotility, **S**clerodactyly and **T**elangiectasia.)

AKT Paper 4: Questions

1) *Calculating cardiovascular risk*

A 55-year-old woman comes to your surgery worried about her strong family history of cardiovascular disease. You check her blood pressure, do some bloods and calculate her cardiovascular risk.

At what level of risk would she benefit from starting a statin?

A 10-year absolute risk of 10%
B 10-year relative risk of 10%
C 10-year absolute risk of 20%
D 10-year relative risk of 20%
E None of the above

2) *Cardiac failure*

A 51-year-old woman with known chronic heart failure attends your surgery. She has just been discharged from hospital following a deterioration of her right heart failure. She has recovered well. She wants to know what early warning signs she can look for to prevent the same thing happening again.

Which is the best EARLY indicator of deterioration in chronic heart failure?

A Shortness of breath
B Ankle swelling
C Night wakening
D Weight gain
E Chest pain

3) *Red flag signs in back pain*

A 27-year-old joiner presents with a 2-week history of lower back pain.

Which of the following is MOST likely to point towards serious pathology?

A Inability to work
B Previous episode of low back pain
C Previous history of testicular cancer
D Sciatic nerve pain
E Pain worse on bending forward

4) *Childhood measles*

A 5-year-old boy presents with his mum who is worried that her son might have measles.

Which of the following is NOT a feature of measles?

A Conjunctivitis
B Pain
C Rash
D Coryza
E Cough

5) *Informed consent in a young person*

A 15-year-old girl attends your surgery requesting the contraceptive pill. She is in a consensual relationship with a boy her own age and has been using condoms until recently. She does not wish her parents to know she is going on the pill.

When deciding if it is appropriate to prescribe, which of these is NOT part of the Fraser guidelines?

A The young person understands the advice being given
B The medical practitioner should respect the young person's wish not to involve their parents and it is inappropriate to try to persuade them otherwise
C It is likely that the young person will begin or continue having intercourse with or without treatment/contraception
D Unless he or she receives treatment/contraception their physical or mental health (or both) is likely to suffer
E The young person's best interests require contraceptive advice, treatment or supplies to be given without parental consent

6) *Erectile dysfunction*

Viagra (sildenafil) can be prescribed by GPs on the NHS and endorsed as 'SLS' to treat erectile dysfunction in men who have which ONE of the following conditions?

A Psychological distress
B Parkinson's disease
C Ischaemic heart disease
D Hodgkin's disease
E Stage 3 chronic kidney disease

7–12) *Contraceptive choices*

For the following scenarios, identify the MOST logical suggestion for contraception:

A Suggest a copper IUCD
B Use a combined pill containing more oestrogen
C Use a combined pill containing more progesterone
D Suggest a progesterone-only pill
E Suggest a Mirena coil
F Suggest levonorgestrel (Levonelle) emergency contraception
G Suggest a parenteral progesterone-only preparation
H Continue current contraception
I Suggest condom use

7) A 27-year-old woman complains of breakthrough bleeding on Microgynon 30. She would like to try an alternative pill. Her smear test, swabs and speculum exam are all normal.

8) An 18-year-old girl would like emergency contraception. She had unprotected sex 4 days ago.

9) A 38-year-old lady complains of unmanageable heavy periods lasting for 2 weeks in the month. She is currently taking the progesterone-only pill. She would like to continue to use contraception.

10) A 17-year-old girl is about to start oral retinoids for severe acne. She has been using condoms reliably up until now. She wants to make sure she does not get pregnant while on the medication.

11) A 28-year-old woman has been on Microgynon 30 for 5 years. She has recently started having migraines with focal neurological symptoms. She would like to continue to take her pill if possible.

12) A 17-year-old student comes to you looking for contraceptive advice. She would like reliable contraception and is concerned that she will struggle to remember to take the pill. Choose TWO of the above most appropriate options to recommend to her.

13) *Hepatitis C diagnosis*
A 20-year-old heroin addict has just discovered his ex-partner is hepatitis C positive. He last had sexual intercourse with her 8 months ago. They regularly shared needles when they were together. He wants tested for hepatitis C.
Which of the following is the best test to identify active hepatitis C infection?

A Liver biopsy
B Polymerase chain reaction for HCV RNA
C HCV antibody testing
D HBV antibody testing
E Polymerase chain reaction for HCV DNA

14) *Treatment of hepatitis C*
A 20-year-old heroin addict whose ex-partner tested positive for hepatitis C 2 months ago has also just tested positive for hepatitis C. He has come today to discuss the possibility of being treated.
All of the following factors are considered appropriate for treatment of hepatitis C EXCEPT:

A Mild disease
B A desire to have treatment
C Continued injection of heroin
D Age under 18
E Severe disease

15) *Power of studies*
Which of the following statements regarding studies is true?

A The null hypothesis states that there is a difference between two groups being studied
B A type I error occurs when the null hypothesis is falsely accepted
C A type II error occurs when the null hypothesis is falsely accepted
D The p value stands for power value
E A p value of 0.05 will occur by chance alone, 1 time in 50

16) *Sensitivity*
The sensitivity of a test is the number of:

A true positives detected by the test divided by the number of all true positives in the population tested
B true negatives detected by the test divided by the number of all true negatives in the population tested
C true negatives detected by the test divided by the total number of false positives in the population tested
D true negatives detected by the test divided by the total number of true negatives in the population tested
E true positives detected by the test divided by the total number of true negatives in the population tested

17) *Type I statistical errors*

A type I statistical error in a study is:

A The null hypothesis is falsely rejected
B The statistical analysis was incomplete or incorrect
C The null hypothesis is falsely accepted
D The formulated study question is irrelevant
E The groups are not adequately randomized

18) *Kawasaki's disease*

A 2-year-old girl presents with fever of 5 days, swollen hands and feet with peeling of the fingers and toes, strawberry tongue, cracked lips, non-tender cervical lymphadenopathy and a polymorphous truncal rash. A diagnosis of Kawasaki's disease is made.

Which TWO treatments should be given to this girl?

A Oral aciclovir
B Oral aspirin
C Oral paracetamol
D IV benzylpenicillin
E IV immunoglobulin

19) *Methotrexate*

Which of the following statements regarding methotrexate is correct?

A Any profound drop in white cell or platelet count calls for immediate reduction of methotrexate dose
B Folinic acid is used to counteract the folate–agonist action of methotrexate and is given 24 hours prior to methotrexate
C It is usually prescribed once weekly at a starting dose of 7.5 mg
D Reporting minor colds and sore throats becomes necessary if lasting more than 5 days
E Patients require weekly full blood count and renal and liver function tests while on methotrexate

20) *Lumbar disc prolapse*

A 29-year-old woman attends your surgery with a 2-day history of severe, sudden onset back pain.

Which of the following is correct regarding lower back pain?

A Lumbar disc prolapse most commonly affects the 30- to 40-year-old age group
B Lumbar spine X-ray is often useful in the acute setting
C Patients with concomitant urinary retention should be referred urgently for spinal decompression
D Physiotherapy is unhelpful
E Two weeks' bed rest is a first line treatment option

21–27) *Benefits*
Match the following scenarios with the benefit they should claim:

A Attendance allowance
B Disabled concessions
C Disability living allowance
D Statutory sick pay
E Incapacity benefit
F Income support
G Child benefit
H Carer's allowance
I Social fund benefits
J Unemployment benefit

21) A 67-year-old woman who struggles with activities of daily living due to osteoarthritis and early Alzheimer's disease. She needs care both day and night.

22) A 19-year-old woman gives up work to care full time for her mum who has end-stage COPD.

23) A 35-year-old labourer suffers a back injury at work and is forced to take a month off to recover.

24) A 29-year-old self-employed plumber injures his back at work. He has to take a month off from work to recover.

25) A 50-year-old woman who is claiming the higher rate of disability living allowance wonders if she might be entitled to help with her council tax.

26) A 45-year-old man whose family is on a low income has to pay for his wife's funeral when his wife dies unexpectedly a few weeks after being diagnosed with ovarian cancer.

27) A 45-year-old woman whose rheumatoid arthritis has progressed such that she cannot walk safely without being accompanied by her husband. He also helps her with washing and dressing.

28) *Branded versus generic prescribing*
Exceptions to generic prescribing include all of the following EXCEPT:

A Antibiotics
B Ciclosporin
C Diltiazem
D Nifedipine MR
E Co-amilofruse

29–33) *Groin lumps*
For each of the clinical examination findings below, select the most likely diagnosis:

A Lymph nodes
B Femoral hernia
C Incarcerated hernia
D Inguinal hernia
E Psoas abscess
F Saphena varix

29) A 45-year-old teacher presents with a groin lump. A small, bluish lump is palpated in the medial aspect of the groin. It transmits a cough impulse. It disappears when the patient lies down.

30) A 65-year-old homeless man attends complaining of swelling in his groin. He says he is suffering from night sweats. On examination, he has bilateral swellings in his groin.

31) A 35-year-old building labourer presents with an uncomfortable groin lump. A lump will be felt above the inguinal ligament against the pulp of your finger when the patient coughs.

32) You see a local homeless man at the local GP out-of-hours service. He travelled to the UK illegally from West Africa. He complains of back pain and is found to be pyrexial. A fluctuant mass is palpated in the groin.

33) An 82-year-old obese woman presents with a mass below the inguinal ligament. It is painless and reducible.

34) *Cleaning contaminated body fluids*

You are working in the out-of-hours service during an outbreak of winter vomiting. You are asked to assist in cleaning where a patient has vomited in the waiting room.

What is the single best cleaning agent for contaminated body fluids on work surfaces?

A Betadine
B Chlorhexidine
C Hypochlorite
D Sodium chloride
E Sodium perborate

35–39) *Analgesia*

For each of the patients below select the single most appropriate form of analgesia from the following list of options:

A Bisphosphonates
B COX-2 inhibitors
C Futuro splint
D Local steroid injection
E Methotrexate
F NSAIDs
G Tramadol

35) A 25-year-old pregnant woman complains of numbness and tingling in the thumb, index and middle fingers of her right hand that is worse at night.

36) A 50-year-old woman with metastatic breast carcinoma complains of headaches.

37) A 55-year-old woman presents with a hot and swollen first metatarsal joint of the big toe. She has had no relief with paracetamol. She has no history of peptic ulcer disease.

38) A 65-year-old woman suffers from disabling rheumatoid arthritis of the hands, wrists and right knee. She has always resisted treatment for her rheumatoid arthritis, preferring to use herbal joint rubs wherever possible. She wants you to prescribe something because she is struggling to cope with the pain. She also has active peptic ulcer disease and heart failure.

39) A 40-year-old carpenter presents with pain on the lateral aspect of his elbow. He reports that the pain is worse when he uses his screwdriver. He is self-employed and feels he cannot stop work. You suspect tennis elbow. Ibuprofen and paracetamol have not been helpful. He would like a more definitive treatment.

40) *Risk factors for osteoporosis*
A 50-year-old woman attends your surgery to discuss the risk of osteoporosis. Her mother died following a hip fracture at the age of 80.
Which of the following is a risk factor for osteoporosis?

A Female African–Caribbean race
B Pakistani ethnicity
C Obesity
D High calcium intake
E High fluoride intake

41–46) UK *childhood immunization schedule*
Match the following sets of immunizations with the age at which they would be expected to be given:

A DTP and IPV in one syringe and MMR in a second
B Td/IPV
C DTP, IPV, Hib in one syringe and MenC in a second
D DTP, IPV, Hib in one syringe, MenC in a second and PCV in a third
E Hib and MenC in one syringe.
F DTP, IPV, Hib in one syringe and PCV in a second
G PCV in one syringe and MMR in a second

Key: DTP, diphtheria, tetanus and pertussis (whooping cough); Hib, *Haemophilus influenzae* type b; IPV, inactivated polio vaccine; MenC, meningitis C; PCV, pneumococcal conjugate vaccine; Td, diphtheria and tetanus.

41) 2 months

42) 3 months

43) 4 months

44) 12 months

45) 13 months

46) 13–18 years

47) *Constipation in children*
A 5-year-old girl presents with her parents due to chronic constipation. This has been a problem for her since weaning. Her
parents have already tried to increase her fibre and fluid intake
but are finding this is making little difference.
Which of the following statements is correct here?

A Rectal examination is indicated to exclude faecal impaction
B Abdominal X-ray must be obtained to exclude pathology
C Lactulose may be safely prescribed
D Dehydration is an uncommon cause of constipation in children
E Left iliac fossa mass is commonly tumour

48) *Cardiopulmonary resuscitation*
In which of the following scenarios, is CPR least likely to be successful in restoring a cardiac output?

A A 24-year-old man whose heart has stopped due to hypothermia.
   He has been suffering from depression and has jumped from a bridge
   into a river.
B A previously well 80-year-old who prior to her sudden unexpected
   collapse, had been fit, well and independent.
C A 60-year-old woman who has suffered from longstanding chronic
   cardiac failure who has been deteriorating over the past month
   at home.
D A 3-year-old child whose heart has stopped due to electrocution.
E A 30-year-old heroin addict whose heart has stopped due to heroin
   overdose.

49) *Scotoma*
A 30-year-old woman presents with sight problems. She states that
her field of vision has gradually reduced over the years. She was
adopted but has recently tracked down her mother who suffers
from retinitis pigmentosa.
**Which of the following scotoma descriptions is most likely to apply
to this patient?**

A Central scotoma
B Centrocaecal scotoma
C Arcuate scotoma
D Scintillating scotoma
E Peripheral ring scotoma

50) *Postnatal depression*
A 26-year-old woman attends for her 6-week postnatal check. She says she has been feeling down since the birth of her child.
Which evidence-based questionnaire is recommended for postnatal depression?

A Beck
B Edinburgh
C Hamilton
D Glasgow
E Zung

51) *Good Medical Practice for GPs*
Which of the following is NOT part of the RCGP guidelines for Good Medical Practice for GPs?

A Working with colleagues
B Health and performance of other doctors
C Teaching, training, appraising and assessing
D Maintaining good medical practice
E Minimize NHS costs by rationing appropriately

52) *NICE guideline on dyspepsia*
A 45-year-old woman attends your surgery with a history of chronic dyspepsia.
Which of the following features do NOT warrant urgent referral for endoscopic investigation?

A Chronic GI bleeding
B Epigastric mass
C Iron deficiency anaemia
D Persistent symptoms despite *H. pylori* testing, treating and acid suppression therapy
E Persistent vomiting

53) *GMS Quality and Framework Payments*
A 60-year-old man has multiple chronic conditions. He looks after himself poorly. He accuses you of only being interested in looking after 'illnesses that earn you money'.
Which of his chronic diseases is, in fact, included in the Quality and Outcomes Framework?

A Chronic liver disease
B Chronic obstructive pulmonary disease
C Psoriasis
D Osteoarthritis
E Allergic rhinitis

54–56) *Hypercalcaemia*
Complete the following algorithm with the appropriate diagnoses

A Dehydration
B Bone metastases
C Cuffed specimen
D Hypoparathyroidism
E Chronic renal failure
F Vitamin D deficiency

Causes of Hypercalcaemia

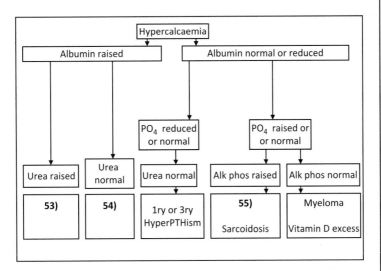

57) *Carr–Hill formula*
The Carr–Hill formula is used to calculate the global sum for practice income.
Which of the following does NOT affect the Carr–Hill formula?

A A high proportion of very old patients
B A high proportion of female patients
C A high proportion of very young patients
D A high list turnover rate
E A high proportion of deprived patients

58) *Faith considerations*

Below is a list of considerations that may apply regarding health-care. To which of the World Faiths do these apply?

- Fasting during Ramadan may be a consideration when planning regular medication. Changes can often be made to limit medications to before dawn and after sundown.
- Appointment times may be required to be made to avoid times of prayer, five times daily.

A Buddhism
B Hinduism
C Islam
D Judaism
E Sikhism

59) *Syringe drivers*

You visit a 70-year-old gentleman who has bronchial carcinoma. He is currently on a number of drugs to control his symptoms. **Which of the following can go into the same syringe as diamorphine?**

A Oramorph
B Chlorpromazine
C Midazolam
D Prochlorperazine
E Diazepam

60–63) *Laxatives*

Match each of the following medications with their mechanism of action:

A Bulk-forming laxatives
B Faecal softeners
C Osmotic laxatives
D Stimulant laxatives
E None of the above

60) Lactulose

61) Arachis oil

62) Ispaghula husk

63) Bisacodyl

64–68) *Diagnosis of falls*
For each of the following clinical scenarios, which is the MOST appropriate diagnosis?

A Vestibular neuronitis
B Aortic stenosis
C Benign paroxysmal positional vertigo
D Carotid sinus hypersensitivity
E Cerebellar syndrome
F Impaired vision
G Ménière's disease
H Parkinson's disease
I Postural hypotension
J Sensory ataxia
K Sick sinus syndrome
L Vasovagal episode

64) A 60-year-old woman present with nausea and vomiting of 3 days' duration. She had a head cold 1 week ago. The nausea is accompanied by severe vertigo. She prefers to lie on her settee with her eyes closed. She has never experienced anything like this before.

65) A 68-year-old gentleman attends your surgery with his daughter. She is concerned because he has had a number of falls over the past 6 months. He feels slowed down and stiff. On examination, he has generalized stiffness and mild cogwheel rigidity. Examination is otherwise normal.

66) A 68-year-old woman presents following recurrent falls. Her son reports that her walking has been odd for the past few months. In particular, he thought she 'stamped about' a lot. On examination, Romberg's is positive. She says she is in good health. She states she used to get 3-monthly injections, but she stopped those years ago because she felt she did not need them.

67) A 17-year-old woman gives blood for the first time. While making her way across the hall to have tea and a biscuit she starts to sweat. She is next aware of being on the floor, surrounded by people. She is very embarrassed by the situation and wants to leave as soon as possible.

68) A 57-year-old man presents with recurrent episodes of dizziness. He finds these are worse in the morning. He had a myocardial infarction 1 year ago and is taking aspirin, isosorbide mononitrate and a beta-blocker.

69) *Level of evidence*

You are reviewing the latest national guidelines on the treatment of otitis media in children. Regarding the use of a new inhaled treatment, the guidelines suggest benefit with a Ib level of evidence.
What does this imply?

A Presence of evidence from a panel of experts
B Presence of at least one experimental trial
C Presence of at least one controlled, non-randomized trial
D Presence of at least one randomized controlled trial
E Presence of meta-analysis

70) *Levels of evidence*

You are reviewing the latest guidelines concerning the treatment of obesity in adults. A new drug treatment is recommended with Grade A evidence.
What does this imply?

A Presence of evidence from a panel of experts
B Presence of at least one experimental trial
C Presence of at least one controlled, non-randomized trial
D Presence of at least one randomized controlled trial
E Presence of benefit in trials direct from the manufacturing drug company

71) *Management of COPD*

A 45-year-old man attends your surgery due to breathlessness on exertion and cough. He is known to have COPD. On performing spirometry, his FEV1 is 30% of predicted.
According to the British Thoracic Society Guidelines for the management of stable COPD, which of the following treatments is advised here?

A Regular combined inhaled short-acting β_2-agonists and anticholinergics and 30 mg oral prednisolone for 2 weeks
B Regular combined inhaled short-acting β_2-agonists and anticholinergics, corticosteroid trial and antibiotic therapy
C Regular inhaled short-acting β_2-agonists and regular inhaled anticholinergics, corticosteroid therapy and long-acting β_2-agonists
D Regular inhaled short-acting β_2-agonists or regular inhaled anticholinergics and consider corticosteroid therapy
E Theophylline and long-term oxygen therapy

72) *Specialist referral in COPD*
Specialist referral in the management of COPD is required in all of the following situations EXCEPT:

A Cor pulmonale
B Oxygen therapy
C Family history of α_1-antitrypsin deficiency
D Diagnosis under the age of 50
E Bullous lung disease

73) *Long-term oxygen therapy in COPD*
You are seeing a 78-year-old woman for her COPD review. Her daughter thinks she might benefit from home oxygen, though the patient herself is resistant as she does not want to be 'confined to the house'.
Which of the following would suggest that referral for oxygen therapy might be appropriate?

A FEV1 59%
B Presence of peripheral oedema
C More than two exacerbations per year
D Her husband required oxygen therapy for his COPD before he died
E Oxygen saturations on air of 95%

74) *Treatment of scabies*
A mother attends the out-of-hours service with her two children. She complains of intense itching throughout the whole family. She thinks they may have caught scabies from another household where her daughter attended a sleepover party 3 weeks ago. On examination, the mother has widespread excoriations with evidence of burrows between her fingers.
What is the most appropriate recommendation?

A Apply malathion 0.5% preparation over entire body after a hot bath and wash off after 12 hours. Repeat in 1 week's time
B Apply benzyl benzoate over the whole body; repeat without bathing on the following day and wash off 24 hours later. Repeat for up to 3 consecutive days
C Apply permethrin 5% dermal cream over whole body and wash off after 12 hours. Repeat in 1 week's time
D Prescribe ivermectin as a single dose of 200 µg/kg by mouth
E Apply carbaryl lotion over whole body after hot bath and wash off after 24 hours. Repeat once a week for 3 consecutive weeks

75–81) *Distribution graphs*

Match the following distribution graph descriptions:

A Bimodal
B Low mean. Low variance
C High mean. High variance
D Low mean. High variance
E High mean. Low variance
F Negatively skewed distribution
G Normal distribution
H Positively skewed distribution

75) Mean > median > mode

76) Mode > median > mean

77) Mean = median = mode

78) A tall, thin, symmetrical graph with a high peak

79) A wide, squat, symmetrical graph with a low peak

80) A graph charting the mean blood pressure for a population of 1000 patients

81) A graph with two peaks

82–87) *Antiplatelet agents*

For each of the following clinical situations, select the most appropriate treatment according to current guidelines:

A No antiplatelet treatment required
B Aspirin only
C Clopidogrel only
D Dipyridamole only
E Aspirin and clopidogrel in combination
F Aspirin and dipyridamole in combination
G Clopidogrel and dipyridamole in combination
H Warfarin

82) To prevent a cardiovascular event in a patient who has reduced walking distance due to peripheral vascular disease.

83) A 56-year-old man is discharged from hospital following a first episode of acute coronary syndrome. His hospital investigations showed a non-ST elevation myocardial infarction (NSTEMI).

84) A 60-year-old woman who is admitted to hospital with a first episode of chest pain. She is diagnosed with an ST elevation myocardial infarction and is thrombolysed on admission.

85) A 50-year-old man who has a bare metal stent inserted following coronary angiography for unstable angina.

86) A patient presents with symptoms classic of transient ischaemic attack. You start medication prior to them being seen at the rapid access cerebrovascular clinic.

87) A 57-year-old woman who would like advice on whether she should take an antiplatelet. Following investigation, her cardiovascular risk factor calculation gives her a 10-year absolute risk of 15%.

88–91) *Dermatological conditions*
For each of the following scenarios, select the MOST likely diagnosis:

A Body lice
B Contact dermatitis
C Eczema
D Leukoplakia
E Lichen planus
F Lichen sclerosus
G Psoriasis
H Scabies

88) A 40-year-old hairdresser presents with an itchy rash on her inner wrists. The lesions are small reddish-purple papules and appear in linear form. She thinks it is due to a reaction to chemicals at work and is considering changing jobs.

89) An 80-year-old female resident of a nursing home presents with an itchy generalized rash over her body, which spares her face. She reports that the itching is worse at night. On examination she has an itchy papular rash with isolated vesicles on her hands. She has no skin signs elsewhere.

90) A 50-year-old man presents with a mouth ulcer he cannot get to heal. On examination, he has a white lesion on the undersurface of his tongue. The white marks cannot be scraped off. He is a heavy smoker.

91) A 28-year-old female who smokes 20 cigarettes per day presents with linear plaques and palmar pustulosis.

92) *Peripheral nerve injury*
A 45-year-old man attends with left leg weakness. On examination, he has weakness of the hamstrings on the left side. He also has sensory loss below the knee, sparing the medial border of his foot. **What is the likely nerve injury here?**

A This does not correspond to a single peripheral nerve lesion
B Tibial nerve
C Sciatic nerve
D Common peroneal nerve
E Cauda equina lesion

93–97) *Karyotypes*
Match the following karyotypes with their associated conditions:

A Trisomy 13
B Trisomy 18
C Trisomy 21
D 45X
E 47XXX
F 47XXY
G 46X
H 46Y
I 46XXX

93) Down's syndrome

94) Klinefelter's syndrome

95) Edwards' syndrome

96) Patau's syndrome

97) Triple X syndromes

98–100) *Cancer incidence*
For both male and female patients in the UK, put these cancers in order of incidence, starting with the MOST frequently diagnosed:

A Bladder carcinoma
B Breast carcinoma
C Colorectal carcinoma
D Lung carcinoma
E Non-Hodgkin's lymphoma
F Prostate carcinoma

98) Most commonly diagnosed

99) Second most commonly diagnosed

100) Third most commonly diagnosed

AKT Paper 4: Answers

1) C 10-year absolute risk of 20%
Become familiar with cardiovascular risk calculators and how to convey risk to patients.

2) D Weight gain
We should encourage daily weighing, as a 2 kg weight gain is a useful early sign of fluid retention. Reporting such gains can avoid hospitalization due to shortness of breath later.

3) C Previous history of testicular cancer
Previous history of cancer is a red flag sign. Mechanical back pain is often recurrent and is a major cause of loss of work. Red flag signs for back pain are as follows:
- non-mechanical pain
- thoracic pain
- fever, weight loss or ill health
- known previous cancer, HIV, steroids
- cauda equina symptoms: bowel or bladder dysfunction; saddle anaesthesia
- age of onset <20, >55.

4) B Pain
Malaise would be a feature of measles, but not pain as such. Measles is uncommon now so it is worth revising the features, which comprise a 2–4-day prodrome of fever, cough, conjunctivitis and coryza (3Cs). There is then a generalized rash for 3 or more days which tends to appear first at the hairline, spreading downwards, becoming confluent. The rash fades to leave brown discolouration and sometimes fine desquamation. Koplik's spots are red spots with a blue/white central spot. They are found on the buccal mucosa, classically opposite the second molars. If measles is suspected, contact Public Health and discuss local testing methods (oral liquid sample or swab).

5) B The medical practitioner should respect the young person's wish not to involve their parents and it is inappropriate to try to persuade them otherwise
The Fraser guidelines focus on the desirability to have parents involved and apply specifically to giving contraceptive advice to under 16s. 'Gillick competence' is used to identify children under 16 who have legal capacity to consent to medical treatment. The Fraser guidelines should be fulfilled prior to prescribing contraception to an under 16 year old.
1. The young person understands the advice being given.
2. The young person cannot be convinced to involve parents/carers or allow the medical practitioner to do so on their behalf.

3. It is likely that the young person will begin or continue having intercourse with or without treatment/contraception.
4. Unless he or she receives treatment/contraception their physical or mental health (or both) is likely to suffer.
5. The young person's best interests require contraceptive advice, treatment or supplies to be given without parental consent.

6) B Parkinson's disease
Viagra is licensed for ED in men who have DM, MS, Parkinson's, poliomyelitis, prostate cancer, severe pelvic injury, single gene neurological disease, spina bifida, spinal cord injury, on renal dialysis, kidney transplant, or who have had radical pelvic surgery or prostatectomy. It can be given by specialist centres, but not by GPs, in cases without the above conditions where the patient is suffering severe distress as a result of impotence. It is contraindicated in recent stroke, unstable angina and myocardial infarction.

7) C Use a combined pill containing more oestrogen
In breakthrough bleeding, first exclude a cervical cause and check compliance. Try increasing the progestogen content. If this is unsuccessful, then increase oestrogen content too. Due to the risks associated with the oral contraceptive pill, always use the lowest possible oestrogen content pill. Microgynon 30 remains the most common oral contraceptive pill.

8) A Suggest a copper IUCD
A copper IUD is licensed for emergency contraception up to 5 days. Can usually be fitted without difficulty even in a nulliparous woman. Levonelle is licensed up to 72 hours after unprotected sex.

9) E Suggest a Mirena coil
Mirena coil is now the first line of treatment for menorrhagia if contraception is required.

10) G Suggest a parenteral progesterone – only preparation
This would include Depo-Provera or Implanon. Oral retinoids are known teratogens. Pregnancy must be excluded and reliable long-term contraception initiated prior to starting them. In nulliparous women, Depo-Provera or Implanon is ideal.

11) D Suggest a progesterone – only pill
Migraine with focal symptoms is an absolute contraindication for the combined pill due to increased risk of stroke.

12) I Suggest condom use
Remember the role of condoms in preventing sexually transmitted infection.

13) B Polymerase chain reaction for HCV RNA

HCV antibody testing identifies if a patient has been exposed to hepatitis C. HCV RNA PCR identifies if the infection is active. Hepatitis C is an RNA virus. Acute infection is usually asymptomatic but jaundice and malaise may occur. The incubation period is between 2 and 25 weeks (average 8 weeks). Usually antibody positive 3 months from acute infection although in some cases it is up to 6 months before a patient becomes antibody positive. Around 25% of those infected with the virus will clear the virus at the acute stage.

14) D Age under 18

NICE guidelines advocate treatment for all who desire it, including continued heroin injection and mild disease. Previous guidelines advocated treatment in severe disease only. Treatment is pegylated interferon and ribavirin. This clears the virus in 40–60% of those treated. Virus clearance means undetectable viral levels 6 months after stopping treatment.

15) C A type II error occurs when the null hypothesis is falsely accepted

The *null hypothesis* states that there is no difference in outcome in two groups being studied – usually a case group and a control group.

A *type I error* in a study is where the null hypothesis is falsely rejected or, to put it another way, to state a significant difference between the items studied which has occurred by chance or by bad study design. An example of this would be the first studies published linking MMR vaccination to autism. Dozens of subsequent studies have shown no such association. We can therefore conclude that, in the first study, a type I error occurred.

The *p-value* is a measure of how much evidence we have against the null hypothesis. By convention, $p < 0.05$ is used to represent statistical significance. When a p value is not < 0.05, it is either because there is no statistical difference between the two groups, or because the numbers in the study were not large enough. However, $p < 0.05$ will occur naturally by chance alone, 1 time in 20. For a study to be adequately powered to draw significant conclusions, large numbers of study subjects are usually required.

A *type II error* is when the null hypothesis is falsely accepted, i.e. to see no difference between the study and control groups where there is in fact a difference. An example of this would be COX-2 inhibitors. Until recently, there were no concerns about cardiovascular risks associated with COX-2 inhibitors. Subsequently, further study and re-analysis of previous data showed that there appears to be an increased risk of cardiovascular events using COX-2 inhibitors. In initially thinking there was no such association, a type II error occurred.

When carrying out a study, high numbers of patients are required to ensure a meaningful or true result. This is referred to as 'power'. If a trial is underpowered, the numbers are too small to detect a small difference between the two treatments or groups being studied.

16) A The number of true positives detected by the test divided by the number of all true positives in the population tested

Sensitivity = the number of true positives detected by the test divided by the true positives in the population tested. A 70% sensitivity means that 70% of those with the disease will test positive and the other 30% will test negative.

Specificity (option B) = true negatives detected by the test divided by the true negatives in the population tested. A 60% specificity means that 60% of those who do not have the disease will correctly test negative and the other 40% will incorrectly test positive. Sensitivity and specificity are absolute properties of a test. They do not change for a test regardless of how common or uncommon a disease is.

17) A The null hypothesis is falsely rejected

The null hypothesis is that there is no difference between the two groups. A type I error is when the null hypothesis is falsely rejected. This means that the study finds a difference that does not really exist, i.e. the result is a statistical fluke. The conventional cut-off for statistical significance is $p = 0.05$, or a 1 in 20 chance. Hence if 20 trials were conducted, it would be expected to get one that was 'positive' by chance alone.

18) B Oral aspirin

E IV Immunoglobulin

Kawasaki's disease is a systemic vasculitis. Young children suspected of having this disease should be referred urgently for prompt treatment to prevent coronary artery damage and give symptomatic relief, ideally, before 10. They should have IV immunoglobulin and aspirin.

Remember the Kawasaki 5C mnemonic: Children; Cervical lymph nodes; Conjunctivitis; Cutaneous (rash); Coronary microaneurysms.

19) C It is usually prescribed once weekly at a starting dose of 7.5 mg

Methotrexate is usually given once weekly for the treatment of leukaemia, psoriasis and rheumatic disease. Any drastic drop in white cell or platelet count calls for immediate **withdrawal** of methotrexate and administration of supportive therapy. Folic acid is given once weekly **after** the dose of methotrexate to counteract the folate–antagonist effect of methotrexate. The Commission on Human Medicines has recommended a new warning label on methotrexate after numerous medication errors and overdosing by patients taking their dose daily. Patients are advised to report **all** symptoms and signs suggestive of infection, especially sore throat. Blood tests are recommended before treatment is commenced, weekly until therapy stabilizes and thereafter every 2–3 months. Methotrexate may induce pneumonitis, which is treated with steroids.

20) C Patients with conconitant urinary retention should be referred urgently for spinal decompression

Prolapsed lumbar disc is most common in the 20–30-year-old age group. The discs involved are L4/5 or L5/S1. Early X-rays are unhelpful. Lumbar disc prolapse is a clinical diagnosis. Urinary retention is a red flag sign indicating cord compression. 90% of patients are better within 6 weeks and 95% by 3 months. Gentle early mobilization and physiotherapy with analgesia is advocated to aid recovery and maintain function. The Cochrane Review from 2001 concluded that bed rest was not effective and may be deleterious.

Examination should include movement in all directions in the back, neurological examination of the lower limbs and straight leg raise to assess the sciatic nerve.

21) A Attendance allowance
A tax-free, non-means-tested allowance for a person over the age of 65 with a severe physical or mental disability requiring care during the day or both day and night. Conditions should have lasted over 6 months, unless a terminal illness is involved where life expectancy is less than 6 months. Lower rate for daytime care only or at higher rate for day and night care.

22) H Carer's allowance
Allowance for a carer older than 16 who spends more than 35 hours a week caring for someone receiving attendance allowance or middle/high rate care level of Disability Living Allowance.

23) D Statutory sick pay
Paid by employers to employees who have made adequate national insurance contributions. Lasts up to 28 weeks.

24) E Incapacity allowance
This is paid at three different rates (short-term at lower rate, short-term at higher rate and long-term after 1 year) to a person unfit for work on medical grounds and who has paid NI contributions. Can be paid instead of statutory sick pay for those who are self-employed.

25) B Disabled concessions
This includes assistance with travel, council tax relief, exemption from road tax, free dental care, free glasses and free prescriptions and social services assistance.

26) I Social fund benefits
This will pay for cold weather, funeral and maternity expenses, i.e. exceptional, one-off expenses.

27) C Disability living allowance
Equivalent to attendance allowance but for under 65s. Has a care component, paid at three rates, for help with washing, dressing and hygiene. Also has a mobility component, paid at two rates for poor walking ability. Disability should last for more than 3 months.

Income support is a benefit for those with low income, with little savings, and doing less than 16 hours paid work per week. *Child benefit* is a non-means tested benefit for households with children under 16.

The *Oxford Handbook of General Practice* has a helpful summary section on the benefit system.

28) A Antibiotics

Working in the NHS and being responsible for the public purse, it is wise to prescribe generically wherever possible. There are some exceptions to this rule of thumb, however. Drugs with a narrow therapeutic window such as lithium, carbamazepine, phenytoin and ciclosporin are exempt from generic prescribing as minor variations in bioavailability between brands might make a big difference to the pharmacodynamics of the drug. Other reasons to prescribe by brand include modified-release preparations such as nifedipine and diltiazem and multi-drug formulations such as co-amilofruse. In both of these cases, minor variations in manufacturing could make a significant clinical difference.

29) F Saphena varix

Saphena varix may also be associated with a bluish tinge to the skin; however, this is not always present.

30) A Lymph nodes

Bilateral swellings point toward lymph nodes being a cause. The differential diagnosis here includes lymphoma, HIV and tuberculosis.

31) D Inguinal hernia

Clinically, direct and indirect herniae are difficult to distinguish. This may only be established intraoperatively. Herniae should be assessed and managed conservatively or referred for surgery.

32) E Psoas abscess

This man has spinal tuberculosis (Pott's disease) which has formed an abscess that has tracked to the psoas muscle. Spinal TB is uncommon in the western world, but is increasing in frequency.

33) B Femoral hernia

A femoral hernia will lie below the inguinal ligament. Remember the inguinal ligament runs from the pubic tubercle medially to the anterior superior iliac spine laterally. Femoral herniae are more common in women; inguinal herniae are more common in men. Femoral herniae are at higher risk of strangulation than inguinal herniae.

34) C Hypochlorite

In general practice and out-of-hours services there are no on-call domestic service to clean unexpected spills of bodily fluids. Medical and nursing staff are expected to be aware of infection control procedures.

According to the Health Protection Agency, vomit should be cleaned with a dilute bleach solution (0.1% hypochlorite) to ensure destruction of the Norwalk-like virus, which is transmitted through the vomit of an infected individual. Sodium perborate is an antiseptic mouthwash and is similar to hydrogen peroxide and chlorhexidine. In a winter vomiting outbreak, hands should be decontaminated by general detergent hand washing followed by alcohol hand rub.

35) C COX-2 inhibitors
Carpal tunnel syndrome is associated with pregnancy. Night splints are the most appropriate treatment here. Surgery would clearly be inappropriate in pregnancy.

36) G Tramadol
Strong opioid analgesia is indicated here though which would be first choice is a matter of local protocol and personal experience. If cerebral metastases and raised intracranial pressure are suspected, oral dexamethasone is the medication of first choice.

37) F NSAIDs
Gout is the diagnosis here. Any NSAIDs (diclofenac, indometacin or naproxen) may be prescribed. Allopurinol started in an acute attack will exacerbate symptoms. Colchicine can be used second line but has diarrhoea and vomiting as side effects.

38) F NSAIDs
COX-2 inhibitors are contraindicated in patients with heart failure. NSAIDs could be cautiously prescribed with a proton pump inhibitor to prevent gastrointestinal bleed. Patients with this degree of disabling rheumatoid arthritis are usually under secondary care. Disease-modifying agents such as methotrexate or leflunomide should be considered as well as symptomatic treatment.

39) D Local steroid injection
Remember tennis elbow affects the lateral epicondyle of the elbow, golfer's elbow affects the medial epicondyle. Tennis elbow can be treated conservatively with NSAIDs and rest. Steroid injection can speed recovery. Physiotherapy and epicondylar brace can be considered though are not usually used first line.

40) B Pakistani ethnicity
Risk factors for osteoporosis include:
- Asian
- Caucasian
- family history
- female
- excess alcohol
- excess caffeine
- low oestrogen in women
- low testosterone in men
- underweight
- smoking

- overexercising, i.e. exercise-induced amenorrhoea
- late menarche
- early menopause
- corticosteroids.

Factors protective against osteoporosis include:

- male
- female African–Caribbean race
- high intake of calcium and fluoride
- obesity
- weight-bearing exercise.

41) F DTP, IPV, Hib in one syringe and PCV in a second

42) C DTP, IPV, Hib in one syringe and MenC in a second

43) D DTP, IPV, Hib in one syringe, MenC in a second and PCV

44) E Hib and MenC in one syringe

45) G PCV in one syringe and MMR in a second

46) B Td/IPV

This could also be asked in an algorithm format.

UK childhood immunization schedule	
2 months	2 injections: DTP/IPV/Hib+PCV
3 months	2 injections: DTP/IPV/Hib+MenC
4 months	3 injections: DTP/IPV/Hib+MenC+PCV
12 months	1 injection: Hib/MenC
13 months	1 injection: PCV+MMR
3 yrs 4 mths	2 injections: DTP/IPV+MMR
13–18 yrs	1 injection: Td/IPV

In addition, BCG and Hep B vaccines are given at birth to groups at higher risk of tuberculosis and hepatitis B. You may prefer to learn the immunization schedule by remembering the course schedule for each individual vaccine; for example, PCV is given at 2, 4 and 13 months.

47) C Lactulose many be safely prescribed

First line therapy should be dietary manipulation with increased fibre and fluid intake. Lactulose with or without additional senna or sodium picosulfate can be used as a first line medication in children with chronic constipation. *Note:* If there is a suspicion of faecal impaction, lactulose should not be used. It is rare to subject a child to a PR examination. Firm stool should be palpable during abdominal examination. Abdominal X-ray is not indicated, as clinical diagnosis should be clear. Dehydration is a common cause of constipation in children. Parents often report the problem being worse in summer. Lower gastrointestinal tumour is extremely rare in children.

48) C A 60-year-old woman who has suffered from longstanding chronic cardiac failure who has been deteriorating over the past month at home
Although some of these scenarios are likely to be seen in routine general practice, it is important to understand the appropriateness of CPR when discussing resuscitation decisions with patients. On average, only 17% of patients who have resuscitation successfully carried out in the community survive to be discharged from hospital. The figures are much lower in patients with serious underlying conditions. Age is no barrier to CPR, although in general it is less likely to be successful in the elderly. The presence of a serious underlying condition is a much better predictor of poor outcome.

49) E Peripheral ring scotoma
In retinitis pigmentosa, an autosomal dominant cause of blindness, pigment is gradually deposited on the retina, beginning at the peripheries, resulting in a ring scotoma progressing to tunnel vision. The term scotoma refers to an area of visual loss, which is surrounded by normal vision. The area of loss corresponds to the area of pathology in the retina. The blind spot is a physiological scotoma.
- *Central scotoma*: macula, e.g. age-related maculopathy.
- *Centrocaecal scotoma*: nerve (e.g. toxic neuropathy); enlargement of blind spot towards central vision.
- *Peripheral ring scotoma*: retinitis pigmentosa.
- *Arcuate scotoma*: also occurs as an extension of the blind spot but is arcuate in shape. Sometimes called 'Seidel's scotoma', this occurs in glaucoma.
- *Scintillating scotoma*: area of 'fuzzy vision' which can occur as migraine aura.

50) B Edinburgh
The Edinburgh Postnatal Depression Questionnaire is a validated and widely used scale to assess for postnatal depression. The others are self-assessment questionnaires for depression, but the Edinburgh scale is most commonly used in the postnatal period.

51) E Minimize NHS costs by rationing appropriately
The principles of good medical practice do not generally refer to rationing as this would assume that all UK doctors work within the NHS. Rationing applies in a different manner in private practice. This document shares some similarities with the GMC's Good Medical Practice:
- *good clinical care*: provide the best possible care
- *maintaining good medical practice*: striving to continually improve
- *relationships with patients*: communicating effectively with patients to build relationships
- *working with colleagues*: promoting positive communication and working environment

- *teaching, training, appraising and assessing*: as part of continually maintaining knowledge and skills
- *probity*: practising with honesty and openness
- *health and performance of other doctors*: all doctors have a responsibility to report when they are concerned about their own or their colleagues' fitness to practise.

52) D Persistent symptoms despite *H. pylori* testing, treating and acid suppression therapy
Consider urgent referral for patients presenting with persistent vomiting and weight loss, unexplained weight loss or iron deficiency anaemia, as well as those with unexplained worsening of dyspepsia combined with Barrett's oesophagus, known dysplasia, atrophic gastritis or intestinal metaplasia, or peptic ulcer surgery over 20 years ago. Refer urgently for endoscopy patients aged 55 years and over with unexplained and recent onset dyspepsia alone.

53) B Chronic obstructive pulmonary disease
Although there are financial incentives involved in the targets for each clinical indicator in the Quality and Outcomes Framework (QOF), the purpose behind this contract is to ensure high-quality, evidence-based patient care. An up-to-date set of QOF targets is available via the Department of Health website. Your practice manager will be well versed in these. This is a useful tutorial subject. Chronic kidney disease, but not chronic liver disease, is included in the clinical indicators list.

54) A Dehydration

55) C Cuffed specimen

56) B Bone metastases
The other options are causes of hypocalcaemia. Interpretation of blood results is a common multiple choice question.

57) B A high proportion of female patients
Factors used in calculating the Carr–Hill formula include the following:
- age/sex adjustments – the very young and the very elderly, requiring the most care
- nursing and residential homes – generate a disproportionately high workload
- list turnover – lists with a high turnover generate a higher workload
- rurality – rural practices have higher costs due to a practice population spread over a much wider area
- staff market forces factor (MFF) – staff costs will vary throughout the country, with higher wages in London for example.
 The Carr–Hill formula is calculated in a different way in the various countries of the UK.

58) C Hinduism

People of any faith or culture will vary in how they carry out customs. It is important to discuss relevant issues with individual patients.

59) C Midazolam

Oramorph is an oral medication and not appropriate for parenteral administration. Chlorpromazine, prochlorperazine and diazepam are not suitable for administration in a driver because of local skin irritation. According to the *BNF*, the following can be mixed with diamorphine:

- cyclizine
- dexamethasone
- haloperidol
- hyoscine butylbromide
- hyoscine hydrobromide
- levomepromazine
- metoclopramide
- midazolam.

  For further details on compatibilities, refer to the Palliative Medicine Handbook: http://book.pallcare.info.

60) C Osmotic laxatives

61) B Faecal softeners

62) A Bulk-forming laxatives

63) D Stimulant laxatives

- Bulk forming laxatives
  - Ispaghula husk
  - Methylcellulose
  - Sterculia
- Stimulant laxatives
  - Bisacodyl
  - Dantron (Co-danthramer/Co-danthrusate)
  - Glycerol suppositories
  - Senna
  - Sodium picosulfate
- Faecal softeners
  - Arachis oil
  - Liquid paraffin
- Osmotic laxatives
  - Lactulose
  - Macrogols (Movicol)
  - Magnesium salts
  - Rectal phosphate enemas (Fletchers' phosphate enema)
  - Rectal sodium citrate (Microlette Micro-enema)

64) A Vestibular neuronitis

Vestibular neuronitis is an acute, severe vertigo. Nystagmus and vomiting accompany it. It occurs following viral infections. It is self-limiting though symptoms can be helped using labyrinthine sedatives, e.g. cyclizine or prochlorperazine. Cooksey–Cawthorne physiotherapy exercises can aid recovery.

65) H Parkinson's disease

First presentation Parkinson's can be subtle. The three primary features are the extrapyramidal features of bradykinesia, rigidity and tremor. The asymmetrical and unilateral onset of resting tremor is probably the single best clinical clue that one is dealing with true Parkinson's disease. In particular, presentations in the elderly can easily be attributed to other causes if a physical examination is not carried out. Drug history may suggest drug-induced Parkinsonism, especially if on antipsychotic medication.

Features of Parkinson's disease include:

- akinesia/bradykinesia – small, shuffling steps
- cogwheel rigidity – rigidity and tremor
- festinant gait – a bent-forward gait with short steps as if trying to catch up with your own centre of gravity
- reduced arm swing
- kinesia paradoxica – the ability to perform faster movement more easily than slower ones.

66) J Sensory ataxia

Sensory ataxia is caused by the loss of proprioception. Its gait tends to involve a high-stepping, stamping, wide-based gait while looking at the ground. The 3-monthly injections suggest previous pernicious anaemia. Chronic B12 or folate deficiency can cause subacute combined degeneration of the cord. This is degeneration of the dorsal columns of the spinal cord, which convey touch, vibration and proprioception. Other causes of sensory ataxia are syphilis and multiple sclerosis.

67) I Vasovagal episode

This is a classic history of vasovagal syncope. Young people are particularly at risk. If any other relevant past medical history had been present, it would have been picked up at screening by the blood transfusion service.

68) I Postural hypotension

Postural hypotension tends to be worse in the morning. All anti-anginals have hypotension as a side effect. Awareness of the cause of the dizziness and behaviour modification may be enough to resolve the problem. If simple measures do not help, the next step would be medication review.

69) D Presence of at least one randomized controlled trial

When guidelines are put together, authors cross-reference their recommendations with the level of evidence that goes along with them. These are as follows:

- Ia – meta-analysis of randomized controlled trials
- Ib – at least one randomized controlled trial
- IIa – at least one well-designed controlled trial which is not randomized
- IIb – at least one well-designed experimental trial
- III – case, correlation and comparative studies
- IV – evidence from a panel of experts

70) D Presence of at least one randomized controlled trial
When guidelines are produced, for each recommendation the level of evidence that led to that recommendation is given alongside it. This is then translated into a 'Grading of recommendation' which can be used very easily when applying the guidelines.
Grading of recommendation

- Grade A: based on evidence from at least one randomized controlled trial (i.e. Ia or Ib)
- Grade B: based on evidence from at least one non-randomized controlled trial (i.e. IIa, IIb evidence) or extrapolated from hierarchy I evidence
- Grade C: based on experimental descriptive studies (comparative, correlation and case-control studies – level III evidence) or extrapolated from level I, II or III evidence)
- Grade D: based on evidence from a panel of experts (i.e. IV).

71) A Regular combined inhaled short-acting β_2-agonists and anticholinergics and 30 mg oral prednisolone for 2 weeks
A very brief summary of the COPD guidelines is as follows:
START   Avoid risk factors, e.g. occupational/smoking AND flu vaccine
ADD   prn short-acting bronchodilator (e.g. salbutamol)
ADD   short-acting bronchodilator and anticholinergic
ADD   regular long-acting bronchodilators (one or more)
ADD   inhaled steroids if repeated exacerbations
ADD   theophylline
ADD   long-term oxygen therapy. Consider surgical options.
These are the bare bones of the guidelines. Where there is flexibility there may be a preference for combined inhalers. There are some major advantages in using combined inhalers in certain patients. When a patient is symptom free, they may not take their steroid 'preventer' inhaler because they feel they do not need it. When wheezing, cough or shortness of breath begins, they reach for their 'reliever inhaler'. Combined inhalers mean patients who would not normally take them get an early dose of inhaled steroid, thereby shortening the exacerbation. Combined inhalers are now included in the guidelines for both asthma and COPD.

72) D Diagnosis under the age of 50
Indications for hospital admission with an exacerbation of COPD

- Marked increase in intensity of symptoms, e.g. sudden onset resting SOB

- severe background COPD
- onset of new physical signs, e.g. cyanosis, peripheral oedema
- failure to respond to initial medical management
- significant comorbidities
- newly occurring arrhythmias
- diagnostic uncertainty
- older age
- insufficient home support
  reasons to consider secondary care in COPD
- long-term oxygen therapy
- commencement or withdrawal of long-term oral steroids
- pulmonary rehabilitation
- surgery
- of course guidelines are just that. Different GPs will have varying levels of comfort with dealing with severe COPD in the community.

73) B Presence of peripheral oedema
The need for oxygen therapy should be assessed in the following:
- all patients with severe airflow obstruction (FEV1 <30% predicted)
- patients with cyanosis
- patients with polycythaemia
- patients with peripheral oedema
- patients with raised JVP
- patients with oxygen saturations ≤92% breathing air.
  Assessment should be considered in patients with moderate airflow obstruction (FEV1 30–49% predicted).

  Overall, in the AKT, respiratory questions are done badly by candidates. Be familiar with the latest guidelines for COPD and asthma. One possible reason for this might be that GP trainees are not having adequate exposure to these patients because of practice nurse input. It would be a good use of time for trainees to carry out a COPD or asthma clinic alongside the practice nurse. Otherwise, familiarize yourself with the commonly used inhalers, where they occur in the guideline algorithms, and their mode of action.

74) C Apply permethrin 5% dermal cream over whole body and wash off after 12 hours. Repeat in 1 week's time
Treat all household members and give clear instructions. Use permethrin as a first line treatment. Use malathion if permethrin is inappropriate. Treatment must be reapplied if hands are washed. It is particularly important to have the webs of the fingers treated. Remember, the itch and rash will last much longer than the treatment and doesn't necessarily indicate failure. Use topical antihistamines and oral antihistamines to deal with this.

75) H Positively skewed distribution

76) F Negatively skewed distribution

77) G Normal distribution

78) E High mean. Low variance

79) D Low mean. High variance

80) G Normal distribution

81) A Bimodal

Normal distribution is the most common curve. It is symmetrical, predictable and normally distributed data are analysed using parametric tests (Mean = Median = Mode).

Non-normal data are skewed, i.e. one tail of the graph is longer than the other. Remember when drawing a skewed graph, the direction of skew refers to the direction of the **longer tail**. In a positively skewed distribution, the tail is extended in the **positive** direction (i.e. to the right) (Mean > Median > Mode). In a negatively skewed distribution, the tail is extended in the **negative** direction (i.e. to the left) (Mode > Median > Mean).

An alternative way to remember this is to always put the three terms in alphabetical order: Mean – Median – Mode.

Remember positive as '>' and negative as '<'. Use whichever works best for you.

Variance is a measure of spread. A wide graph has a high variance; a narrow graph has a low variance.

A bimodal distribution has two peaks; a multimodal distribution has multiple peaks.

Practice sketching the different types of graph to ensure you are familiar with them.

82) B Aspirin only

Patients with peripheral vascular disease should be considered high risk for a cardiovascular event. Use 300 mg aspirin as a loading dose, then 75 mg daily.

83) E Aspirin and clopidogrel in combination

With NSTEMI, NICE guidelines recommend using the aspirin–clopidogrel combination for 12 months before stopping the clopidogrel. Some regions would stop the clopidogrel before this time, between 3 and 12 months. Clopidogrel is usually started with a loading dose of 300 mg, then a maintenance dose of 75 mg.

84) E Aspirin and clopidogrel in combination

For STEMI, use the aspirin–clopidogrel combination for 1 month then stop clopidogrel.

85) E Aspirin and clopidogrel in combination

Use the aspirin–clopidogrel combination for 1 month where a bare stent is present. Continue the combination for 12 months where a drug-eluting stent is present, then stop clopidogrel.

86) F Aspirin and dipyridamole in combination

In TIA and stroke disease, a combination of aspirin and dipyridamole MR should be used for 2 years before the dipyridamole is stopped. If unable to tolerate dipyridamole, use aspirin alone. If unable to tolerate aspirin due to gastric side effects, use aspirin + omeprazole. If unable to tolerate this combination, use clopidogrel alone. The combination of clopidogrel and dipyridamole has not been adequately tested and so is not recommended. Dipyridamole MR is taken 200 mg twice daily.

87) A No antiplatelet treatment required

Primary prevention is recommended for those with a cardiovascular disease risk of ≥20% and for diabetics who are either over 50 or who have had diabetes for more than 10 years. There is no clinical evidence to support the use of any antiplatelet other than aspirin for the primary prevention of cardiovascular disease.

Enteric coated aspirin is not normally recommended to avoid gastric side effects. It is preferable to commence omeprazole.

Always try adding a proton pump inhibitor when facing gastric side effects of antiplatelet drugs before changing the antiplatelet.

Patients may be discharged from hospital on medication which is to be stopped after a period of time; this should be clear on their immediate discharge document. Alternatively, they may be given a separate patient reminder card to clarify duration of treatment.

88) E Lichen planus

This is a very common exam question due to the classic nature of the description. Although the history suggests contact dermatitis, the description suggests otherwise. It is exquisitely itchy with 'pruritic, purple, polygonal papules'. They occur on flexor surfaces, palms, soles and mucous membranes. They exhibit the Koebner phenomenon (lesions occurring along lines of trauma). They may demonstrate Wickham's striae, a fine surface network of white lines. The cause is unknown but likely to be autoimmune. Treat with topical steroid to reduce the itch. Usually self-resolves within a year. Specialist treatment can include PUVA treatment.

89) H Scabies

The generalized nature of the itch and the history of nursing home residence strongly suggest scabies even without classic skin signs.

90) D Leukoplakia

Leukoplakia is a premalignant, white thickening of the oral mucosa and should be biopsied. It is differentiated from candidiasis by the fact that you cannot scrape off the white marks. It is most commonly associated with smoking and alcoholism. Do not confuse with oral hairy leukoplakia, which is associated with immunodeficiency and is not a pre-malignant condition. Similar lesions can occur on the vulva and anus. These are also pre-malignant.

91) G Psoriasis

Psoriasis has a number of classic presentations:

- palmoplantar pustulosis comprises yellow/brown sterile pustules on the palms or soles
- plaque psoriasis is the most common presentation, with well-defined, hyperkeratotic, silvery plaques which demonstrate point bleeding if picked. They occur on extensor surfaces, the sacrum most commonly
- scalp psoriasis is very common and can be mistaken for severe dandruff. The lesions are well demarcated, where dandruff is much more generalized
- flexural psoriasis affects the axillae and submammary areas. Plaques are much more smooth and shiny. It is most common in the elderly
- guttate psoriasis presents as multiple raindrop lesions on the trunk. It can occur following streptococcal throat infection.

92) C Sciatic nerve

There may be a history of back pain here. Sciatic nerve (L4–S2) injury causes weakness of knee flexion and all the muscles below the knee (foot drop). There is loss of sensation below the knee, which spares the medial border of the foot. Common peroneal nerve (L4–S2) injury causes inability to dorsiflex, evert the foot and extend the toes (foot drop). There is sensory loss over the dorsum of the foot. Tibial nerve (S1–S3) injury causes inability to stand on tiptoe, invert the foot or flex the toes. There is sensory loss over the sole.

93) C Trisomy 21

94) F 47XXY

95) B Trisomy 18

96) A Trisomy 13

97) E 47XXX

This is a common multiple choice question.

Revision of karyotypes:

- normal male: 46XY
- normal female: 46XX
- turner's syndrome: 45X (or 45XO)
- triple X syndrome: 47XXX
- klinefelter's syndrome: 47XXY

- edwards' syndrome: Trisomy 18
- down's syndrome: Trisomy 21
- patau's syndrome: Trisomy 13.

98) B Breast carcinoma

99) D Lung carcinoma

100) C Colorectal carcinoma

These incidence statistics are frequently published but are always a few years behind. These statistics are from 2005. To get up-to-date statistics, go to the Cancer Research UK website.

In fact, the most commonly diagnosed cancer is non-melanoma skin cancer, especially basal cell carcinomas. If this is an option in a multiple choice question, it would be most common. Non-melanoma skin cancers are, however, routinely left out of cancer incidence statistics.

Do not confuse incidence statistics with statistics for cancer mortality.

AKT Paper 5: Questions

1–7) *Developmental milestones*
Match the following child development milestones:

A Developing normally
B Delayed gross motor development
C Delayed fine motor and vision development
D Delayed hearing and speech development
E Delayed social development
F Delay in more than one area of development

1) A 4-week-old baby who is gaining weight well. He startles to a loud noise. He is not yet looking at mum while he is breastfeeding.

2) A 23-month-old boy cruises furniture, babbles continuously, feeds himself with a spoon and scribbles with crayons.

3) An 11-month-old girl who can sit with support, but not unsupported, responds to noise but does not yet respond to her own name. She enjoys throwing away toys that are handed to her and enjoys peek a boo.

4) An 18-month-old boy who prefers to eat with his fingers. He cannot master using a spoon to feed himself and makes a terrible mess.

5) An 11-week-old baby who everyone describes as a good baby but mum is concerned her baby doesn't like her. Mum is worried, as the baby has never smiled but instead stares at her intently.

6) A child is about to start school. He will be the youngest in his class and just made the cut-off dates for entry as his birthday is in February. His mum is now having second thoughts about whether or not he is ready to go to school. He can count to 10 and knows some letters. He can draw a picture of a stick figure and appears to make friends easily at nursery. The child himself is anxious about moving up into the 'big school'.

7) A 5-year-old child is getting ready to go to school. Mum attends asking for your advice as her son is still in nappies. He has never once managed to have a dry day or night although he goes to the toilet when asked to. He can dress himself well and knows all of his letters and numbers. He is proud to be going to school but Mum is concerned that she will have to send him to school in nappies.

8–14) *The audit cycle*
Fill in the algorithm of the audit cycle from the following options:

A Set audit standards
B Describe conclusions
C Complete data collection and compare to previous results and standards
D Prepare and plan the audit
E Identify audit criteria
F Complete data collection and compare to standards
G Implement changes

The audit cycle

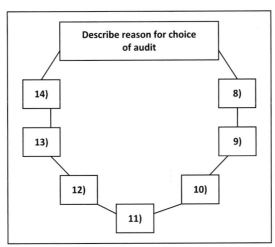

15) *Prophylactic antibiotic in HIV*
Prophylactic antibiotics should be prescribed in HIV-positive patients, if the CD4 count drops below:

A 100 cells/mm^3
B 200 cells/mm^3
C 300 cells/mm^3
D 400 cells/mm^3
E 500 cells/mm^3

16) *Relative risk*

A new class of drug is being tested for rheumatoid arthritis. There are four new drugs in this class. They have severe side effects and are very expensive. Because of this, it is decided that the new drugs will only be incorporated into the local rheumatology clinic's protocols if there is at least a 30% reduction in relapse rate compared to their current favoured treatment.

Based on the following study results, which drug would the clinic take on?

- Monoflex shows a relative risk of relapse of 0.89; $p < 0.0001$
- Duoflex shows a relative risk of relapse 1.77; 95% confidence interval 1.55–2.03
- Triflex shows a relative risk of relapse 0.66; p 0.01
- Quadroflex shows a relative risk of relapse 0.65; 95% confidence interval 0.57–1.3

A Monoflex
B Duoflex
C Triflex
D Quadroflex
E None of the above

17) *Number needed to treat*

The number needed to treat (NNT) is:

A 1/prevalence
B 1/absolute risk
C 1/absolute risk reduction
D 1/relative risk
E 1/relative risk reduction

18–22) *Foot problems*

For each of the following scenarios, choose the most appropriate diagnosis:

A Achilles tendonitis
B Ruptured Achilles tendon
C Plantar fasciitis/bursitis
D Tender heel pad
E Flat feet (pes planus)
F Pes cavus
G Metatarsalgia
H Morton's metatarsalgia (interdigital neuroma)
I Bunion

18) A 35-year-old lawyer attends complaining of foot pain, especially after a long day at work. On examination she is tender between her 3rd and 4th metatarsal heads.

19) A 24-year-old sprinter presents with heel pain. This has come on over some weeks while training for an upcoming national competition. On examination, he has a boggy swelling between his calcaneus and his calf muscle.

20) A 29-year-old hairdresser presents complaining that her shoes do not fit as well as they used to as she has developed a lump at the base of her big toe. She also has pain after a long day at work. She enjoys wearing high fashion shoes and is frustrated at having to wear 'sensible shoes'.

21) A 40-year-old teacher complains of foot pain, especially after a long day at work. It can be particularly painful first thing in the morning, but settles after walking round her bedroom for a few minutes. She always wears flat shoes as she has never found high heels comfortable. On examination, she has inferior heel tenderness.

22) A 39-year-old businessman has injured himself while playing squash. He thought his opponent had kicked him on the back of the heel, but his opponent was at the other side of the court. His left heel is now very painful and he is walking with a limp.

23) *Neuropathic pain*
A 45-year-old man who suffers from longstanding neck and arm pain attends your surgery because he is finding paracetamol and ibuprofen are not helping his pain. His pain is burning in nature and is thought to be neuropathic in nature.
Which would be the next most appropriate drug to recommend?

A Carbamazepine
B Oxycodone
C Gabapentin
D Amitriptyline
E Tramadol

24) *Migraine treatment*
Which two statements regarding treatment for migraines are true?

A Beta-blockers may be used for migraine prophylaxis
B Ergot alkaloids may be prescribed prophylactically
C Aspirin plays no part in migraine analgesia
D Pizotifen may be used for treatment of acute attacks
E 5HT1 antagonists are useful in the treatment of acute attacks

25) *Cradle cap*
A new mum attends your surgery worried about the rash on her newborn baby's head. On examination, the baby has mild cradle cap. The mother is relieved to hear it is nothing serious and asks what she might put on it to take it away.
What would be your first recommendation?

A Betadine shampoo
B Hydrocortisone cream
C Betamethasone cream
D Olive oil
E Cocois scalp ointment

26–31) *Respiratory conditions*
For each of the patients below select the single most appropriate treatment option from the following list of options:

A Amoxicillin
B Clarithromycin
C Losartan
D Prednisolone
E Ramipril
F Salbutamol inhaler

26) A 50-year-old farmer presents with sudden onset of dry cough, fever and shortness of breath. Chest exam reveals basal crackles.

27) A 55-year-old man presents with cough, orthopnoea and paroxysmal nocturnal dyspnoea. On examination, he has a raised JVP and basal rales on auscultation.

28) A 30-year-old man presents with nocturnal cough. His PEFR is 70% of predicted.

29) A 20-year-old man presents with swinging fever, non-productive cough and tender subcutaneous nodules on his anterior legs.

30) A 60-year-old woman on ramipril develops a tickly cough. Chest exam is normal.

31) A 50-year-old homeless man smelling of alcohol presents with fever and a productive cough. Chest exam reveals coarse rhonchi.

32) *Bipolar disorder*
A 30-year-old woman who has suffered from bipolar disorder throughout her 20s. She has found her medication has not been working as well for her over the past year as she has been experiencing hypomania much more frequently. You consider changing her medication.
What would be the most likely SECOND line treatment here?

A Fluoxetine
B Carbamazepine
C Lithium
D Valproate
E Venlafaxine

33–37) *Diagnosis of facial rashes*
For each of the patients below, select the single most appropriate diagnosis:

A Atopic dermatitis
B Cellulitis
C Contact dermatitis
D Dermatomyositis
E Discoid lupus erythematosus
F Impetigo
G Perioral dermatitis
H Psoriasis
I Rosacea
J Seborrhoeic dermatitis

33) A 4-year-old girl returns from nursery with a superficial erythematous rash with a golden-coloured crust around her nose, cheeks and mouth. She is otherwise well. Her mother is concerned about her ability to return to nursery.

34) A 20-year-old woman presents with a burning, itchy rash around her mouth. The eruption spares the skin around the vermilion border of her lips. She has been trying to cover it up with makeup.

35) A 4-month-old baby boy presents with an itchy red rash over his cheeks. His mother suffers from asthma. His mum has been trying to treat it by applying Sudocrem but does not think it is helping.

36) A 40-year-old woman reports facial flushing. On examination she has erythema, papules, pustules and telangiectasia on the nose and cheeks. The facial flushing is made worse by alcohol and sun exposure.

37) A 20-year-old woman presents with several months of facial rash. It started out with polymorphic, red scaly plaques and progressed to follicular plugging, scarring and hypopigmentation. The rash is made worse by sun exposure.

38) *Mental Capacity Act*
You are involved in the care of a 50-year-old lady who has early onset rapidly progressive dementia. She is considering signing Power of Attorney over to her sister rather than her husband. You are concerned that she may not be competent to make this decision any longer.
Which of the following is NOT a principle to be used when referring to the Mental Capacity Act?

A Capacity should always be assumed until proven otherwise
B Always give a patient enough time and opportunity to demonstrate capacity before concluding capacity is not present
C Patients are not entitled to make unwise and unsafe decisions for themselves
D Decisions made for persons without capacity should always be done in that person's best interests
E Decisions made on behalf of patients without capacity should be carried out with least restriction to the patient

39) *Risk of deliberate self harm*
The mother of a 19-year-old man calls the surgery because she is worried about her son. He has not come out of his room for 4 days and has been increasingly reclusive for the past 3 months. He has consistently refused to see the doctor despite his mother's begging.
When assessing this young man, which of the following is the strongest indicator of ongoing suicide risk?

A Evidence of general self-neglect
B Lack of remorse regarding his violent behaviour to his ex-girlfriend
C Morbid jealousy
D Past history of violence with alcohol or drugs
E Persisting denial of responsibility

40) *Breast cancer referral guidelines*

According to the NICE Cancer Referral Guidelines for Suspected Cancer (June 2005), the following clinical features warrant urgent referral to breast clinic EXCEPT:

A A 22-year-old woman presents with bilateral painful breasts
B A 30-year-old woman presents with a discrete mass persisting after next period
C A 20-year-old woman presents with spontaneous right-sided blood-stained nipple. She has no family history of breast cancer
D A 35-year-old woman has persistent right nipple eczema unresponsive to treatment
E A 50-year-old man with a left-sided firm, subareolar mass

41) *ESR*

A 65-year-old woman presents with myalgia, especially in her upper arms. The serum full blood count is normal and the ESR comes back as 40 mm/h.

The next step should be:

A Arrange for CXR and AXR
B Commence oral corticosteroids
C Reassurance
D Refer for temporal artery biopsy
E Take blood for CRP as it is more sensitive

42–47) *Evidence-based management of hypertension*

For each of the following patients, identify the MOST appropriate antihypertensive drug:

A ACE inhibitor
B Alpha-blocker
C Angiotensin II receptor antagonists
D Beta-blocker
E Calcium antagonist (dihydropyridine)
F Calcium antagonists (rate-limiting)
G Thiazide diuretic

42) A 75-year-old man with a history of gout is noted to have persistent BP >170/80 over 3 months.

43) A 50-year-old African–Caribbean man requires antihypertensive therapy.

44) A 70-year-old man with a history of prostatism has a persistent BP >170/100.

45) A 55-year-old man has a history of heart failure and requires antihypertensive therapy.

46) A 60-year-old woman on ramipril complains of persistent tickly cough.

47) A 65-year-old man with a history of angina is noted to have persistently elevated BP.

48–52) *Squint*
Match the following definitions with the correct type of squint:
A Esotropia
B Exotropia
C Latent squint
D Paralytic squint
E Pseudosquint

48) A 5-year-old boy presents because his parents think he might have a squint. His left eye is turned inward.

49) An 8-year-old girl presents with her parents who think she might have a squint. Her right eye is turned out.

50) A child whose diplopia is most marked when trying to look in the direction of the pull of the affected muscle.

51) A newborn baby presents with his parents. They are worried he might have a squint. On examination the baby has prominent epicanthic folds. Corneal reflections are symmetrical.

52) A 10-year-old girl presents with her parents who are worried she might have a squint. On examination, movement of the covered eye demonstrates a squint as the cover is removed during the cover test.

53–57) *Drug treatment in symptomatic heart failure*

Complete the gaps in the algorithm below which shows NICE guidance for treatment of symptomatic heart failure.

A   Start ACE inhibitor and titrate upwards
B   Add digoxin
C   Add spironolactone
D   Add beta-blocker and titrate upwards
E   Add diuretic

Management of chronic heart failure in adults in primary and secondary care. (Reproduced by kind permission of National Institute for Clinical Excellence. July 2003.)

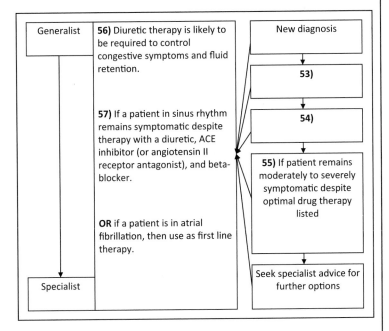

58) *Immunization*

Which one of the following statements regarding immunization is correct?

A   Anaphylactic reaction to egg ingestion contraindicates influenza and yellow fever vaccines
B   Anaphylactic reaction to egg ingestion contraindicates MMR vaccine
C   A personal or family history of inflammatory bowel disease contra-indicates MMR vaccine
D   Children with acute febrile illness should be encouraged to have vaccinations as planned
E   Multiple live vaccines should not be given together

59–64) *Hormone replacement therapy*
For each of the patients below select from the following list of options the SINGLE most appropriate treatment:

A Combined oestrogen/progesterone
B Continuous combined HRT
C Oestradiol patches 50 μg
D Oestradiol pessary
E Raloxifene
F Tibolone

59) A 50-year-old woman requests 'no period' HRT. She is 1 year post-menopausal and also reports low libido and low mood.

60) A 60-year-old woman complains of atrophic vaginitis.

61) A 55-year-old woman requests HRT for hot flushes. She has had a hysterectomy.

62) A 50-year-old woman requests HRT but she does not want to see the return of her periods. She is 1 year postmenopausal.

63) A 60-year-old woman noted to have a kyphotic spine requests HRT. She is not suffering from any menopausal symptoms but she is concerned about osteoporosis.

64) A 40-year-old woman is confirmed to have premature menopause with elevated serum LH and FSH levels.

65) *Symbols used in the British National Formulary (BNF)*
While looking up a medication in the *BNF*, you notice the following symbol: ▼.
What does this symbol mean?

A The drug in question is not for prescription on the NHS
B The drug is subject to prescription under the Misuse of Drugs Act
C This drug is a prescription-only medicine
D There has been limited experience of use of this drug and the CHM requests that all suspected adverse reactions be reported
E This drug is considered by the Joint Formulary Committee to be less suitable for prescribing

66–71) *Postpartum contraception*

Match the following clinical scenarios with the appropriate timing of introduction of contraception after giving birth:

A Immediately
B Day 21
C 4 weeks
D 6 weeks
E 8 weeks
F Delayed until after baby's first birthday

66) A 35-year-old female decides she would like the progestogen-only pill form of contraception. She intends to breastfeed. She has no contraindications to the POP.

67) A 25-year-old female would like the Depo-Provera injection. She intends to breastfeed and has no contraindications to injectables.

68) A 44-year-old female would like sterilization after the birth of her 6th child.

69) A 40-year-old female would like the Mirena IUS fitted after the birth of her 3rd child.

70) A 30-year-old female would like to start Microgynon after giving birth. She intends to bottle-feed and has no contraindications to the COC.

71) A 31-year-old woman has used a diaphragm all of her adult life for contraception. She would like to go back to this form of contraception.

72) *Anthrax*

Which three statements are true concerning anthrax?

A CXR findings are classic for anthrax
B Flucloxacillin is the antibiotic of choice
C Contacts of exposed individuals require prophylaxis
D ID50 is the dose required to infect 50% of exposed individuals
E It is not a notifiable disease

73–79) *Role of committees*

Match the following roles with the correct respective committee:

A CHI
B Clinical Governance
C GMC
D GPC (GMSC)
E LMC
F NCAA
G NICE
H PACT

73) It is the sole negotiating body with the Department of Health and is a standing committee of the BMA and represents all GPs in the UK.

74) It is a statutory body of locally elected GPs who meet monthly locally and annually at a national conference.

75) This analyses prescribing patterns and cost data for each practice and compares them with other practices in the area.

76) This committee oversees the quality of clinical governance and of services. It was established in April 2000 and reviews all types of organizations (e.g. GP practices, hospitals, primary care trusts) regarding their quality of services to patients.

77) This produces and disseminates clinical guidelines to promote cost-effective therapies and uniform clinical standards. It covers guidance on health technology, clinical management of specific conditions, and referral guidelines from primary to secondary care.

78) This is an initiative of the White Paper *The New NHS* and is a framework to improve patient care through high standards, personal and team development and cost-effective, evidence-based clinical practice.

79) This authority assesses a doctor's performance rapidly to avoid years of suspension during an enquiry.

80) *Dianette oral contraceptive pill*
A 30-year-old woman requests a prescription for Dianette for contraception.
Select the SINGLE correct answer regarding this prescription:

A As Dianette is also used to treat acne, the patient will be charged private prices
B Is contraindicated as a form of contraception in diabetic patients
C The prescription must be handwritten
D The prescription should contain the female sign
E This pill comes in a 28-day pack

81) *Breaking confidentiality*
A court order for release of a patient's medical records without the patient's written consent is called:

A Order of determination
B Order of disclosure
C Order of discovery
D Order of public interest
E Order of release of medical records

82–85) *Hypersensitivity reactions*
Match the following disorders with their appropriate hypersensitivity reaction type:

A Type I hypersensitivity
B Type II hypersensitivity
C Type III hypersensitivity
D Type IV hypersensitivity
E Type V hypersensitivity

82) Extrinsic allergic alveolitis

83) Asthma

84) Transfusion reactions

85) Graves' disease

86–88) *Vertigo*
For each of the following clinical scenarios, select the MOST likely diagnosis:

A Migraine
B Ménière's disease
C Benign paroxysmal positional vertigo
D Acoustic neuroma
E Vestibular neuronitis

86) A 50-year-old woman attends with episodes of vertigo, vomiting and pain in the right ear. These attacks have happened on three separate occasions, each a few months apart. On examination during an attack, she has horizontal nystagmus and reduced hearing on the affected side. What is the most likely diagnosis?

87) A 30-year-old woman attends with a 2-week history of dizziness, falling to the ground and vomiting. The onset was very sudden but has gradually improved over the 2 weeks. Her balance remains poor. There is no problem with her hearing.

88) A 40-year-old man presents with recurrent episodes of dizziness. They last only seconds but occur frequently with sudden changes in posture. They occur particularly when he turns over in bed.

89) *Autoantibodies in gastrointestinal disease*
While reviewing blood results in your practice, you come across a test positive for anti-gliadin antibodies.
With which disorder is this most closely associated?

A Pernicious anaemia
B Primary biliary cirrhosis
C Autoimmune hepatitis
D Rheumatoid arthritis
E Coeliac disease

90) *Falls*
You see an 80-year-old patient who is rarely at the practice but who used to see a now retired partner. She is usually fit and well but has been falling more recently. She is worried that she might break a hip. Her medications include amitriptyline, diazepam, temazepam, bendroflumethiazide, atenolol, aspirin and simvastatin.
Which of the following is most likely to reduce her falls?

A Stop aspirin
B Stop simvastatin
C Reduce to four or fewer medications
D Stop amitriptyline
E Stop bendroflumethiazide

91) *Sterilization*

When counselling couples requesting referral for sterilization, which of the following is TRUE?

A Female sterilization has a lower complication rate than male sterilization
B Can be considered to be reversible
C Reversal of sterilization can usually be carried out on the NHS if required
D Male sterilization is the single most reliable form of contraception available
E If a woman becomes pregnant following a tubal sterilization, there is an increased risk of ectopic pregnancy

92) Regarding sterilization, which of the following, DOES NOT increase the likelihood of regret?

A Where the male partner is under 25
B Where the female partner is reaching the end of her reproductive life
C Where the couple already have one child
D Where a vasectomy is carried out during a partner's unplanned pregnancy
E Sterilization at the time of termination of pregnancy

93) *Peripheral nerve lesions*

A 39-year-old woman attends with a longstanding hand problem. She feels she has a weakness of opening her fist. On examination she has a wrist drop and loss of sensation over the dorsum of her hand.

What is the nerve affected here?

A Radial nerve
B Ulnar nerve
C Brachial plexus outflow
D Sciatic nerve
E Median nerve

94) *Antidiabetic agents*

A 50-year-old woman is noted to have persistently raised fasting blood glucose level >7 mmol/L. She is diagnosed with type II diabetes. She is worried about putting on further weight as her BMI is already 31. She works as a bus driver and is worried about hypoglycaemic episodes.

What is the most appropriate first line medication here?

A Metformin
B Gliclazide
C Insulin
D Acarbose
E Rosiglitazone

95) *Sexually transmitted infections in pregnancy*
An 18-year-old woman attends your surgery. She is 25 weeks pregnant. She wants to discuss testing with you because she thinks she may have contracted a sexually transmitted infection.
Which of the following is NOT commonly associated with complications in pregnancy?

A Genital herpes
B Chlamydia
C Gonorrhoea
D Bacterial vaginosis
E Human papilloma virus (HPV) infection

96) *Hypercalcaemia*
Which of the following is NOT a cause of hypercalcaemia?

A Hyperparathyroidism
B Hypothyroidism
C Milk–alkali syndrome
D Sarcoid
E Squamous cell carcinoma

97) *Type II diabetes*
A 60-year-old man presents to your surgery. He complains of feeling tired all the time and has a strong family history of type II diabetes.
Which of the following is NOT associated with a first presentation of type II diabetes?

A Non-healing ulcer in the foot
B Having to get up more frequently in the night to urinate
C Weight loss
D Weight gain
E Ketones in the urine

98–100) *Drug side effects*
Match the following side effects with the drug with which they are classically associated:

A Atenolol
B Carbamazepine
C Cimetidine
D Clozapine
E Isoniazid
F Rifampicin
G Sildenafil
H Tetracycline
I Tricyclic antidepressants

98) Orange–red tears

99) Neutropenia

100) Bronchoconstriction

AKT Paper 5: Answers

1) C Delayed fine motor and vision development
Babies will very quickly show evidence of some vision by staring at faces looking at them or by looking at mum while breastfeeding. No discernible evidence of vision should be a warning sign.

2) B Delayed gross motor development
Children would be expected to walk between 10 and 15 months with walking backwards at 12–22 months.

3) F Delay in more than one area of development
A child of this age should be sitting without support and should recognize his own name.

4) A Developing normally
Children of this age will often prefer using their fingers when they can. A child would be expected to use a spoon by $2\frac{1}{2}$ years. Confidently but appropriately reassuring anxious parents is an important skill.

5) E Delayed social development
An 11-week-old baby should be smiling by now. Mean age is around 5 weeks to smile.

6) A Developing normally
There is no obvious developmental reason to stop him from going to school, but at the younger end of the class it is a personal, parental decision when to send him to school. Advise his parents to ask the nursery teachers' opinion of his readiness for primary school. It is normal for children to be a little anxious about the move.

7) E Delayed social development
A school-aged child might be expected to have the occasional accident but would be expected to be largely dry through the day.
     Developmental milestone questions can be difficult because children vary so widely in their development. In addition, sets of milestones available in textbooks can appear to be very different. For the purposes of memorizing milestones, it is easiest to memorize the **latest** likely age of reaching a milestone. Remember that this will be significantly different to the average age of acquiring skills, but is the more useful piece of information to have at your fingertips when assessing a child in a developmental clinic. Alternatively, you might want to memorize a set of milestones for each age. As the Royal College use the *Oxford*

Handbook of General Practice as the primary source, this is the best set of milestone guidelines to use:

Gross motor development

- lifts head momentarily while lying face down – from birth
- head lag evident – up to 6 weeks
- rolls over – up to 18 weeks
- moro reflex – present from birth. Disappears – up to 6 months
- can be pulled to sit – up to 6 months
- sits with support – up to 6 months
- bears weight on legs – up to 7 months
- sits without support – up to 8 months
- crawls – up to 9 months
- can hold head in line with body when suspended ventrally – up to 10 months
- gets to sitting position – up to 11 months
- pulls to standing – up to 10 months
- walks holding onto furniture – up to 13 months
- walks alone – up to 15 months – bottom shufflers later
- jumps with both feet together – up to 20 months
- walks backwards – up to 22 months
- runs – up to 2 years
- pedals tricycle – up to 3 years
- kicks a ball – up to 24 months
- stands on one foot for 1 second – up to $3\frac{1}{4}$ years
- walks heel-to-toe – up to $5\frac{1}{4}$ years.

Fine motor development and vision

- stares – from birth
- loses primitive grasp reflex – up to 12 weeks
- palmar grasps – up to 6 months
- transfers hand to hand and mouths object – up to 8 months
- fixes and gazes on small objects – up to 8 months
- follows fallen toys – up to 8 months
- casts (throws) – up to 15 months
- delicate pincer grasp – up to 18 months
- bangs bricks together– up to 13 months
- scribbles – up to 24 months
- Builds a tower of 3–4 bricks – up to 24 months
- builds a tower of 8 bricks – up to $3\frac{1}{2}$ years
- copies a cross – up to $4\frac{1}{2}$ years.

Hearing and speech

- startles to loud noise – from birth
- quietens to sound – up to 2 weeks
- vocalizes – up to 6 months
- polysyllabic babbling – up to 10 months
- laughs – up to 5 months

- responds to own name – up to 8 months
- uses mama and dada appropriately – up to 20 months
- uses three additional words – up to 21 months
- points to eyes, nose and mouth – up to 23 months
- obeys simple instructions – up to $2\frac{1}{2}$ years
- puts two words together – up to 24 months
- gives first and last name – up to 4 years
- speaks grammatically – up to $4\frac{1}{2}$ years.

Social behaviour and play

- social smiling – up to 10 weeks
- puts everything into mouth – up to 8 months
- hand and foot regard – up to 8 months
- peek-a-boo – up to 10 months
- uses spoon to get food into mouth – up to $2\frac{1}{2}$ years
- explores environment – up to 20 months
- takes off shoes and socks – up to 20 months
- puts on clothes without supervision – up to $3\frac{1}{2}$ years
- dry in the day – up to 4 years
- comforts friends in distress – up to 5 years.

Alternatively, memorize red flag warning signs:

- at any age: maternal concerns; parental report of a regression in skills previously acquired
- at 10 weeks: no smiling
- at 6 months: persistent primitive reflexes; persistent squint; hand preference; little interest in people toys or noises
- at 10–12 months: no sitting; no double syllable babble; no pincer grasp
- at 18 months: not walking independently; fewer than 6 words; persistent mouthing or drooling
- at $2\frac{1}{2}$ yrs: no 2–3 word sentences
- at 4 yrs: unintelligible speech.

8) E Identify audit criteria

9) A Set audit standards

10) D Prepare and plan the audit

11) F Complete data collection and compare to standards

12) G Implement changes

13) C Complete data collection and compare to previous results and standards

14) B Describe conclusions

The eight-stage audit cycle (from the RCGP Condensed Curriculum Guide)

1. Describe the reason for choice of audit, considering the potential for change and relevance of the audit to the practice.
2. Identify the audit criteria, ensuring the criteria chosen are relevant to the audit subject and are justified by relevant evidence.
3. Set the audit standards; this involves setting appropriate targets and a suitable timescale.
4. Prepare and plan the audit, recording evidence of teamwork and discussion where appropriate.
5. Complete the first data collection, comparing the results against the standards.
6. Implement the changes to be evaluated, with examples described.
7. Complete the second data collection and compare the results with the first data collection and the standards.
8. Describe the conclusions, including any barriers to change and a summary of the issues learned.

15) B 200 cells/mm^3
Prophylaxis against opportunistic infections with reducing CD4 counts:
- <200 cells/mm^3 – at risk from *Pneumocystis jiroveci* (formerly *P. carinii*). Prescribe co-trimoxazole
- <100 cells/mm^3 – at risk from toxoplasmosis. Prescribe co-trimoxazole
- <50 cells/mm^3 – at risk from *Mycobacterium avium intracellulare*. Prescribe azithromycin. Highly active retroviral therapy (HAART) is normally started at a CD4 count of <350 cells/mm^3.

16) C Triflex
- Monoflex shows a reduction in relapse. This is highly statistically significant but not as good as the 30% the clinic is looking for
- Duoflex shows a statistically significant increase in relapse rate so would be rejected
- Triflex shows a relative risk of relapse of 0.66; this is more than a 30% improvement ($p = 0.01$). Statistical significance is arbitrarily set at $p < 0.05$ and so this is statistically significant
- Quadroflex shows a relative risk of relapse that is good enough but the 95% confidence intervals cross 1, so this is not statistically significant

17) C 1/absolute risk reduction
The NNT is the number of patients needed to take a treatment in order to prevent one event; for example, the number of patients needed to be treated with simvastatin to prevent one myocardial infarction. NNT statistics are often easier to express to patients than absolute and relative risks statistics.

18) H Morton's metatarsalgia (interdigital neuroma)
The pain is due to entrapment of the interdigital nerve between the metatarsal heads, usually due to wearing of high-heeled shoes. Presents with pain and paraesthesia on walking. Can be managed conservatively with steroid injection, or, less commonly, surgically with excision of the neuroma. Advice regarding shoes is essential.

19) A Achilles tendonitis
Usually an overuse injury causing a painful swelling of the Achilles tendon. It is a common athletics injury. Treat with rest, non-steroidal analgesia and heel raise shoe inserts. Physiotherapy and steroid injections into the surrounding tissue may also be helpful.

20) I Bunion
Hallux valgus (bunion) is lateral deviation of the big toe at the MTP joint. Can be caused by osteoarthritis or, in young people, by wearing pointed or high-heeled shoes where the shoes rub on the first MTP joint. Commercial pads are available to relieve the rubbing. Shoe advice is essential. Surgery may be considered in severe deformity. Hallux valgus is the term used to describe an abnormally positioned big toe where the joint at the base of the big toe bulges. The big toe points inward. A bunion is a painful swelling of the bursa that occurs at the base of the big toe because of the hallux valgus.

21) C Plantar fasciitis/bursitis
Inflammation of the plantar fascia, which runs in a band along the foot arch, can be stretched and irritated by flat shoes. It is a common condition in hill walkers. Commercial arch supports are available. Arch support, soft heels pads and heel support can be helpful. Achilles tendon stretching exercises may be helpful. Non-steroidal analgesia and steroid injection may be necessary though most settle down with conservative treatment in around 6 weeks. Being over 40 and overweight are also risk factors.

22) B Ruptured Achilles tendon
Ruptured Achilles tendon presents much more acutely than Achilles tendonitis. The mechanism of injury tends to be an abrupt change in speed or direction such as is required in golf or squash, resulting in a sudden pain in the back of the heel. Patients often report that they thought they had been kicked or stamped on only to turn round and find nobody there. A gap can be felt where the tendon is ruptured. On examination there is a loss of plantar flexion and the patient cannot

stand on tiptoes. Urgent referral is required for surgical repair or plaster immobilization to aid healing of the tendon.

23) D Amitriptyline
Neuropathic pain does not tend to respond well to standard analgesics, including strong opioids. The starting dose of amitriptyline should be 10 mg nocte and increased slowly up to 75 mg if necessary. Anticonvulsants such as carbamazepine, phenytoin, sodium valproate, clonazepam and gabapentin are second line drugs. Tramadol and oxycodone are opioid analgesics for nociceptive pain. Topical capsaicin (chilli extract cream) has been used for neuropathic pain. It has a burning sensation on initial use but encourage patients to persevere through this as it settles quickly.

24) A Beta-blockers may be used for migraine prophylaxis
Serotonin agonists (i.e. sumatriptan, naratriptan and rizatriptan) are used for the treatment of acute attacks. Ergot alkaloids (i.e. ergotamine) should never be used prophylactically; their use acutely is limited by many side effects – GI upset and muscle cramps. Pizotifen is useful for the prevention of migraines. Other medications used for prophylaxis include beta-blockers, sodium valproate and topiramate, and an unlicensed use for tricyclic antidepressants (e.g. amitriptyline). Remember the simple analgesics. Many patients manage their migraines adequately with aspirin, paracetamol or ibuprofen at the first sign of an attack. This can be supplemented with an antiemetic such as domperidone. Triptans are 5HT1 *agonists* (not antagonists) and are used in the acute treatment of attacks.

25) D Olive oil
For a mild rash, no treatment may be required though most mothers prefer to treat it for cosmetic reasons. Scaling may be removed with olive oil or baby oil which they may have in the house anyway. The *BNF* also suggests coconut oil application. Capasal shampoo (coconut oil, coal tar and salicylic acid) is indicated for cradle cap. In severe cases, 1% hydrocortisone cream may be indicated. Betadine shampoo and Cocois scalp ointment are not recommended in children under 2 and 6, respectively.

26) D Prednisolone
This farmer may have extrinsic allergic alveolitis. This is a hypersensitivity to various organic dusts. Treatment is removal of allergen, oxygen, IV hydrocortisone and oral prednisolone.
   Extrinsic allergic alveolitis has different names depending on the cause:
- farmer's lung: reaction to spores of thermophilic actinomycetes – *Micropolyspora faeni* or *Thermoactinomyces vulgaris* from wet hay
- bird fancier's lung: reaction to avian antigens from feathers and faeces, especially budgerigars and pigeons

- maltworkers lung: Reaction to *Aspergillus clavatus* from malt and mouldy hay
- mushroom worker's lung: reaction to thermophilic actinomycetes spores: *Micropolyspora faeni* in mushroom mould
- bagossis: reaction to *Thermoactinomyces sacchari* in sugar cane processors.

27) E Ramipril
This man is presenting with signs of heart failure and would benefit from an ACE inhibitor. Medications to consider include ACE inhibitors, diuretics, digoxin, beta-blockers, oral nitrates, hydralazine and spironolactone.

28) F Salbutamol inhaler
This man would benefit from a trial of salbutamol. On a first presentation, more information is required to establish a diagnosis. This may be a wheeze caused by infection or allergy.

29) D Prednisolone
Acute sarcoidosis presents with erythema nodosum, joint pain and swinging fever. Chest X-ray shows bilateral hilar lymphadenopathy. Gradual onset sarcoidosis will present with shortness of breath on exertion, tiredness, dry cough and weight loss. The pathology of sarcoidosis involves non-caseating granuloma in any organ and so symptoms are wide ranging. Patients are treated with steroids. Azathioprine, methotrexate and chloroquine are used as steroid-sparing agents.

30) C Losartan
Losartan is an angiotensin II receptor antagonist. Tickly cough is a well-known side effect of ACE inhibitors such as ramipril, in which case angiotensin II receptor antagonists may be substituted. When learning about classes of drugs for any condition, it is wise to learn the names of some of the drugs in each class so you can adequately identify them.

31) B Clarithromycin
Homeless people are at high risk of atypical pneumonia. If the infection does not clear, he may need investigation to exclude tuberculosis.

32) B Carbamazepine
Although it should be clear, make sure you read the question carefully as you may be asked the **second** or **first** line treatments for a condition. Lithium is usually the first line treatment, and carbamazepine the second line treatment for bipolar disorder. Other drugs which can be used second line are valproate or olanzapine. Although there are a few second line treatments, your choice should be clear from the options given. If not, choose the **best** of the options you have been given.

For example, valproate is an inappropriate choice in a woman of child-bearing age when other alternatives are available, so carbamazepine is the best choice here. Benzodiazepines can be used short term to help agitation and overactivity in stressful situations but is not appropriate for long-term treatment. If an antidepressant is to be used, SSRIs are most likely to be useful. Tricyclic antidepressants are contraindicated in patients with a history of manic symptoms.

33) F Impetigo
This is a classic description of impetigo which is caused by *S. aureus*. Most nurseries exclude children, as it is very contagious, until cleared. Can be treated with topical fusidic acid with oral flucloxacillin or erythromycin.

34) G Perioral dermatitis
Perioral dermatitis commonly affects young women and seems to be triggered by the use of steroid cream on the face. Stopping all creams and cosmetics on the face for 3 months can treat it. Tetracycline antibiotics can be used for treatment as in acne.

35) A Atopic dermatitis
Family history of atopy makes an atopic diagnosis much more likely in this child. Remission occurs by 15 years old in 90%. Treat with regular emollients and steroid creams during flares.

36) I Rosacea
Rosacea consists of erythema and pustules, primarily over the nose and cheeks. Most common in middle-aged men. Contrary to popular belief, it is not caused by alcoholism. This myth grew up due to alcohol making the rash more prominent in people with the condition. Patients may need to be reassured about this. Treatment is with topical or systemic antibiotics such as metronidazole or tetracycline.

37) E Discoid lupus erythematosus
Remember that discoid lupus is an entirely separate condition from systemic lupus. Lesions are sun-sensitive, red and well-defined with scales and keratin plugs. It is a cause of scarring alopecia and loss of skin pigmentation. Treat with steroids and sunblock.

38) C Patients are not entitled to make unwise and unsafe decisions for themselves
In fact, it is a principle of the Mental Capacity Act that competent patients are entitled to make any decision they wish, including those which appear unwise and unsafe decisions for themselves. A straightforward example of this is the unwise decision many people make daily to smoke, or consume large amounts of alcohol. Adults with capacity are entitled to make that decision.

The five principles of the Mental Capacity Act

1. Capacity should always be assumed. A patient's diagnosis, behaviour or appearance should not lead you to presume capacity is absent.
2. A person's ability to make decisions must be optimized before concluding that capacity is absent. All practicable steps must be taken, such as giving sufficient time for assessments; repeating assessments if capacity is fluctuating; and, if relevant, using interpreters, sign language or pictures.
3. Patients are entitled to make unwise decisions. It is not the decision but the process by which it is reached that determines if capacity is absent.
4. Decisions made for people lacking capacity must be in their best interests.
5. Such decisions must also be the least restrictive options for their basic rights and freedoms.

39) A Evidence of general self-neglect
Self-neglect is the strongest evidence here of depression and risk of deliberate self-harm or suicide. Other risk factors include male sex, history of deliberate self-harm, alcohol or drug use, and history of severe mental illness. The other options in this question are indicators of potential risk of violence to others.

40) A A 22-year-old woman presents with bilateral painful breasts
Cyclical breast pain can be treated by reassurance and simple analgesia for the most part. If severe, stop the combined contraceptive pill, consider danazol or bromocriptine. Refer if not resistant to treatment.

Conditions requiring referral

- any new discrete lump
- new lump in pre-existing nodularity
- asymmetrical nodularity that persists at review after menstruation
- abscess
- cyst persistently refilling or recurrent cyst
- pain:
  - if associated with a lump
  - intractable pain not responding to reassurance, simple measures such as wearing a well-fitting bra and common drugs
  - unilateral persistent pain in postmenopausal women.
- nipple discharge in women under 50 with:
  - bilateral discharge sufficient to stain clothes
  - bloodstained discharge
  - persistent single duct discharge.
- all women aged 50 and over
- nipple retraction or distortion, nipple eczema
- change in skin colour.

41) C Reassurance
Calculation of predicted value

- men – ESR given by age in years divided by 2
- women – ESR given by age in (years + 10) divided by 2
- the upper limits of normal for ESR = (10 + age) divided by 2. This woman's ESR is normal but you may wish to repeat it in 6 months if symptoms persist. Alarm bells should ring if the ESR was >100 mm/h. Causes of elevated ESR include rheumatoid arthritis, infection, malignancy, connective tissue disorders (giant cell arteritis), sarcoidosis and renal disease. Appropriate interpretation of ESR is essential because of the risks associated with taking steroids in inappropriately diagnosed polymyalgia rheumatica.

42) E Calcium antagonist (dihydropyridine)
Treat an over-75 with a thiazide diuretic or a calcium channel blocker. As a thiazide may exacerbate gout, a calcium channel blocker is the best choice here.

43) G Thiazide diuretic
This question is perhaps slightly unfair because you could legitimately use a calcium channel blocker or a thiazide. Thiazide would probably be used first line due to reduced cost and track record in black people.

44) B Alpha-blocker
This question demonstrates that guidelines are just that – guidelines. In this circumstance, an alpha-blocker can serve the dual purpose of treating his hypertension and his lower urinary tract symptoms.

45) A ACE inhibitor
ACE inhibitors should be started on diagnosis of symptomatic heart failure.

46) C Angiotensin II receptor antagonists
A dry cough is common with ACE inhibitors. Replace with an angiotensin II receptor antagonist.

47) D Beta-blocker
Beta-blockers are effective at reducing symptoms and preventing cardiovascular events.
You are likely to be familiar with the NICE hypertension guideline shown below. This algorithm applies only if there are no other reasons to start an alternative drug first line.

NICE/BHS Guidelines: Choosing drugs for patients with newly diagnosed hypertension. (Reproduced by kind permission of Management of hypertension in adults in primary care. British Hypertension Society and National Institute of Clinical Excellence. June 2006.)

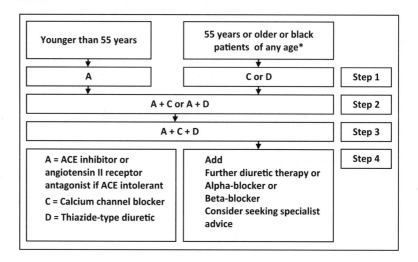

*Black patients are those of African or Caribbean descent, and not mixed race, Asian or Chinese.

48) A Esotropia

Esotropia is another term for convergent squint (strabismus). Amblyopia (lazy eye) may be a problem.

49) B Exotropia

Exotropia is an alternative term for divergent squint. This is often intermittent and tends to occur in older children. Amblyopia is unlikely due to the direction of the squinting (turning) eye. *Note:* An eye that turns upwards is called a hypertropia; an eye that turns downwards is called a hypotropia.

50) D Paralytic squint

Diplopia occurs in the direction of pull of the paralytic muscle. In non-paralytic squint, a full range of eye movement occurs.

51) E Pseudosquint

Pseudosquint commonly presents in young children. Demonstration to parents of symmetrical light reflection on corneas usually provides adequate reassurance (Hirschberg test).

52) C Latent squint
When the affected eye turns when the eyes are open and being used, it is a manifest squint; when the eye turns only when it is covered or shut it is a latent squint.

5% of all 5 year olds will have a squint. All squints require ophthalmological assessment. Management is divided into the 3 'O's: optical, orthoptic and operation. The refractive state of the eyes is determined after use of mydriatic eye drops, and the eyes are inspected to exclude cataract, macular scarring, optic atrophy, retinoblastoma, etc. Spectacles are offered to correct any refractive errors. Orthoptic is the patching of the good eye to encourage use of the squinting (lazy) eye. Finally, resection and recession of the rectus muscles is reserved for cosmesis or alignment.
Other useful ophthalmological terms are as follows:
- hypermetropia – long sight
- myopia – short sight
- astigmatism – the degree of curvature across the cornea or lens differs in the vertical and horizontal planes. The effect of this is that the image becomes distorted vertically or horizontally
- presbyopia – Age-related long sightedness
- amblyopia – lazy eye.

53) A Start ACE inhibitor and titrate upwards

54) D Add beta-blocker and titrate upwards

55) C Add spironolactone

56) E Add diuretic

57) B Add digoxin

58) A Anaphylactic reaction to egg ingestion contraindicates influenza and yellow fever vaccines
Influenza and yellow fever vaccines could potentially cause reactions in susceptible patients. MMR does not have this problem. It is common for patients to ask about personal or family history of various chronic illnesses as a contraindication to vaccination. In fact, patients with chronic illness are often more vulnerable to acute infection, and so vaccination should be encouraged. In children with acute febrile illness, however, vaccination should be delayed until the acute illness is over. Live vaccines should be given either together or separated by at least 3 weeks.

59) F Tibolone

Tibolone has oestrogenic, progestogenic and weak androgenic activity. The androgenic activity has evidence of benefit in low mood and low libido. As a 'no period' HRT, it is inappropriate for use in the perimenopausal period or where the last period was less than 1 year ago due to concerns over increased risk of endometrial hyperplasia.

60) D Oestradiol pessary

Topical oestrogen can improve the symptoms of atrophic vaginitis, whether by pessary or topical cream. It is also used before vaginal surgery for prolapse where there is epithelial atrophy. The smallest effective dose should be used. The endometrial safety of topical oestrogens is uncertain and treatment should be reviewed annually. A short course of oral progesterone once yearly can induce a withdrawal bleed, thus reducing the risk of endometrial hyperplasia.

61) C Oestradiol patches 50 μg

Where the uterus is not present, progesterone is not required to prevent endometrial hyperplasia. Oral oestrogen would be used first line; however, from the options provided, oestradiol patches is the most appropriate.

62) B Continuous combined HRT

Continuous combined HRT has both the oestrogenic and progestogenic components required where the uterus is intact. It is considered safe to use HRT continuously where more than 1 year has passed since the last period.

63) E Raloxifene

Kyphosis strongly suggests the presence of osteoporosis. It is not appropriate to use HRT to treat osteoporosis. Raloxifene is licensed for treatment and prevention of osteoporosis. Vitamin D and a bisphosphonate or raloxifene are appropriate to use in the treatment of osteoporosis.

64) A Combined oestrogen/progesterone

In premature menopause, HRT is essential to prevent bone loss. In women with an intact uterus, both oestrogen and progesterone should be used. Progesterone is given for the last 10–13 days of the cycle. A break from treatment then induces a withdrawal bleed. Treatment should be continued until the age of expected menopause, around 50.

65) D There has been limited experience of use of this drug and the CHM requests that all suspected adverse reactions be reported

Symbols used in the *BNF*

NHS – Not for prescription on the National Health Service (NHS).
CD – Controlled drug. Preparation subject to prescription requirements under the Misuse of Drugs Act.
PoM – Prescription-only medicine. Cannot be bought over the counter.

® – Trade mark.

▼ – Limited experience of the use of this product and all suspected adverse reactions should be reported using the yellow card scheme.

▬ – Considered by the Joint Formulary Committee to be less suitable for prescribing compared to other medications with similar indications.

66) B Day 21
Day 27 is the earliest known day of ovulation following childbirth. It is generally considered that contraception should be used from day 21 following childbirth. If the progesterone-only pill is started after day 21, use barrier contraception for 2 days after starting the pill to ensure adequate protection. This is safe to use in breastfeeding.

67) D 6 weeks
Depo-Provera can be started 5 days after delivery if not breastfeeding. Can carry the risk of erratic, heavy bleeding if started this early postpartum however, especially if breastfeeding. If breastfeeding, delay injection till 6 weeks postpartum. This is to avoid heavy bleeding, and to allow the child's liver enzymes to mature as there is secretion into breast milk.

68) F Delayed until after baby's first birthday
Although theoretically sterilization can take place at any point following childbirth, it is strongly recommended that this be delayed until after the child's first birthday due to increased regret rates if carried out earlier. Also, consider male sterilization as a less invasive procedure.

69) D 6 weeks
Delay insertion of a Mirena IUS until complete involution of the uterus at 6 weeks. Appropriate for use in breastfeeding. Insert at the end of the period if menstruation has returned.

70) D Day 21
There is an increased risk of breakthrough bleeding if started earlier than 21 days. It is recommended that the combined pill not be used until 6 months when breastfeeding. This is because of concerns over hormonal effects on child development and the effect on lactation.

71) D 6 weeks
It is recommended that a woman be re-fitted for a diaphragm after childbirth as the required size is likely to change. For this reason it is recommended that Implanon be inserted 21–28 days after delivery. If inserted after this time, use contraception for 7 days after insertion.

The lactational amenorrhoea method is over 98% effective if the woman is less than 6 months postpartum, is amenorrhoeic and fully breastfeeding on demand. In practice this can be difficult to achieve and women are routinely advised to use additional contraception if wishing not to get pregnant.

72) D ID50 is the dose required to infect 50% of exposed individuals
Anthrax has an incubation period of 1–7 days. It is a Gram-positive rod
diagnosed in cultures from skin or nasal swabs or blood cultures. Three
forms of disease include cutaneous (95%), pulmonary and ingestion.
Cutaneous anthrax results in a black eschar (malignant pustule) 4–9
days after exposure. Oedema, fever and hepatosplenomegaly may also
be present. This form responds to oral ciprofloxacin. Only those
directly exposed to spores should be given 60 days of oral ciprofloxacin
500 mg bd. CXR findings with pulmonary anthrax include widened
mediastinum, lymphadenopathy and haemorrhagic mediastinitis. These
findings can also occur with tuberculosis. The prognosis is poor.

73) D GPC (GMSC)
General Practitioners Committee (General Medical Services
Committee). Represents GPs within the BMA.

74) E LMC
Local medical committee. A body of GPs. Usually operates within
the constructs of the local trust.

75) H PACT
The PACT scheme in England, the Scottish Prescribing Analysis in
Scotland and the Prescribing Audit Reports and Catalogues in Wales.
They include prescribing costs and trends, comparing practices
within the local area.

76) A CHI
Commission for Health Improvement. A government body whose
remit is to ensure quality control within the NHS.

77) G NICE
National Institute for Health and Clinical Excellence. Aims to
produce uniform national, high quality, evidence-based guidelines.

78) B Clinical Governance
Clinical governance is a framework to improve quality within the NHS.
Takes in staff development and improving evidence-based practice.

79) F NCAA
The National Clinical Assessment Authority (NCAA) assesses a
doctor's performance rapidly to avoid years of suspension during
an enquiry.

80) D The prescription should contain the female sign
Dianette cannot be prescribed as an acne treatment on the NHS. If you
do not put the female symbol or at least write 'for coc' on the
prescription, the patient will not be charged NHS prescription costs but

instead private prescription charges. Without the symbol, the prescription indicates a private prescription for use for acne and not an NHS prescription for contraception.

81) C Order of discovery
The phrase covers any situation where a court requests documents which would otherwise be confidential.

82) C Type III hypersensitivity

83) A Type I hypersensitivity

84) B Type II hypersensitivity

85) E Type V hypersensitivity

Hypersensitivity reactions

- Type I hypersensitivity (anaphylactic or immediate): antigen + IgE on mast cells and basophils react. It occurs in asthma, atopy and some acute drug reactions.
- Type II hypersensitivity (antibody-dependent cytotoxicity): cell-bound antigen + circulating IgG or IgM antibody react. It occurs in transfusion reactions, Goodpasture's syndrome, immune thrombocytopenia and rhesus incompatibility.
- Type III hypersensitivity (immune complex-mediated or arthrus reaction): free antigen + free antibody react producing complement activation. Where there is excess exposure to antigen, antigen–antibody complexes at the site of exposure produce disease, e.g. farmer's lung, pigeon and pulmonary aspergillosis.
- Type IV hypersensitivity (cell-mediated or delayed hypersensitivity): antigen with class II MHC (major histocompatibility complex) +memory T-cells react. Reactions take around a day to develop. Occurs in tuberculin testing, contact dermatitis and graft-versus-host reactions.
- Type V hypersensitivity (stimulatory reactions): antibody + cell surface receptor react. Occurs in Graves' disease and thyrotoxicosis.

86) B Ménière's disease
Ménière's disease is caused by distension of the endolymphatic compartment of the inner ear. There is episodic vertigo for hours at a time with sensorineural deafness and a sensation of pressure in the ear, with nystagmus. If unilateral deafness is constant, acoustic neuroma should be excluded via MRI.

87) E Vestibular neuronitis

The sudden onset suggests viral vestibular neuronitis. This tends to be short lived and self-limiting and will resolve gradually over weeks. Treat with rest and antiemetics. With a less sudden onset, consider intracranial tumour.

88) C Benign paroxysmal positional vertigo

Episodes are shorter than in Ménière's disease. Antiemetics are not as helpful as they are in Ménière's. Thought to be caused by otoliths in the labyrinths. Treatment is with Epley's manoeuvre and habituation.

89) E Coeliac disease

Autoantibody results must be interpreted with caution in gastrointestinal disease; these are highly specific but not necessarily highly sensitive.

Autoantibodies in gastrointestinal disease

- anti-gliadin, anti-endomysial antibodies − coeliac disease. Anti-gliadin antibodies should disappear following adequate treatment
- anti-mitochondrial antibodies − primary biliary cirrhosis (+ve in 96%)
- anti-smooth muscle antibodies − autoimmune hepatitis, cryptogenic cirrhosis
- gastric parietal cell antibodies − pernicious anaemia (+ve in 90%)
- intrinsic factor antibodies − pernicious anaemia (+ve in 70%).

90) C Reduce to four or fewer medications

Tapering and stopping benzodiazepines and antidepressant medications can reduce falls. Reducing the number of medications to four or fewer can reduce falls. If postural hypotension is present, stopping atenolol is more likely to be beneficial than stopping bendroflumethiazide.

91) E If a woman becomes pregnant following a tubal sterilization, there is an increased risk of ectopic pregnancy

Male sterilization is a less invasive procedure than female sterilization. Most reversals of sterilization are carried out privately. Implanon is more reliable than male sterilization. Female sterilization has a 0.5% failure rate; male sterilization has a 0.1% failure rate; Implanon has a failure rate of 0.05%.

92) B Where the female partner is reaching the end of her reproductive life

Regret is less likely where either partner is over 35. Regret is more likely where either partner is under 25 or where the couple have fewer than two children. Sterilization during a pregnancy or at the time of delivery should be carried out following assessment by an obstetrician. Usually sterilizations are carried out after a child's first birthday. The emotional nature of termination of pregnancy means it increases risk of regret.

93) A Radial nerve

Radial nerve (C5–T1) injury causes wrist drop and sensory loss over the dorsum of the hand and anatomical snuffbox. Median nerve (C5–T1) injury can cause weakness of thumb flexion and loss of sensation over the thumb, index finger, middle and lateral half of the ring finger. Ulnar nerve (C7–T1) injury causes claw hand deformity and loss of sensation over the medial half of the ring finger and little finger.

94) A Metformin

Metformin is the most common first line agent. It does not cause hypoglycaemia. Diabetic patients who drive will be especially keen to avoid insulin as, for most, it will involve them losing their group II driving licence. Gliclazide and the glitazones can cause hypoglycaemia. Acarbose is rarely used to treat diabetes now. A new class of medications includes drugs such as sitagliptin. These may help prevent type II diabetes patients from gaining weight. They have not yet been added to diabetic guidelines.

95) E Human papilloma virus (HPV) infection

Vaginal discharge, pelvic pain and symptoms of urinary tract infection should be aggressively treated in pregnancy as most infections are associated with increased risk of pregnancy loss or premature labour. Human papilloma virus does not cause cervical or pelvic inflammation and is not associated with complications of pregnancy. Presence of genital herpes at the time of labour may necessitate a caesarean section. Chlamydial conjunctivitis in neonates should be treated aggressively. Chlamydia, gonorrhoea and bacterial vaginosis may cause cervicitis or pelvic inflammation, leading to early labour.

96) B Hypothyroidism

The most common causes of raised calcium in general practice are primary hyperparathyroidism and malignancy. Thyrotoxicosis rather than hypothyroidism can cause hypercalcaemia. This may be associated with osteoporosis. Milk–alkali syndrome results from patients with dyspepsia consuming milk- and alkali-containing antacids, which may reduce the renal excretion of calcium. Sufferers of sarcoid may have high calcium levels. Malignancy is the most well known association with hypercalcaemia.

Revision of types of hyperPTHism

- *Primary hyperparathyroidism*: The circulating level of PTH is inappropriately high. Most patients are hypercalcaemic but may be normocalcaemic if they also have vitamin D deficiency. There is excess production of parathyroid hormone (PTH); although usually from a benign adenoma, this sometimes results from hyperplasia of the parathyroid glands and, in rare cases, a carcinoma. Treatment is usually surgical.
- *Secondary hyperparathyroidism*: This is raised PTH in response to chronic hypocalcaemia or hypophosphataemia, usually due to

renal failure. Serum calcium is low and the parathyroids are hyperplastic. Treat the underlying cause.

- *Tertiary hyperparathyroidism*: This is inappropriately high PTH causing raised calcium levels. It follows prolonged secondary hyperparathyroidism. This is most common in patients with chronic renal failure, especially in dialysis patients, or in chronic malabsorption. The parathyroids are hyperplastic but fail to return to normal once the initiating stimulus is removed. Treatment is usually surgical.

97) E Ketones in the urine

Weight gain and feeling tired all the time is the most common presenting feature of type II diabetes. Obesity is also a major risk factor for developing diabetes. Patients who have been ignoring symptoms of tiredness and polyuria for some time, however, may present with weight loss due to their longstanding feeling of being unwell. Ketonuria is a feature of type I diabetes. Polyuria and polydipsia can occur in both types I and II diabetes and are caused by elevated blood sugar. If the diagnosis is late, the patient may present with symptoms of complications such as ulcers due to peripheral neuropathy, or with symptoms of renal dysfunction.

98) F Rifampicin

99) D Clozapine

100) A Atenolol

Of course it is unreasonable to expect candidates to have memorized the whole of the *BNF* but there may be some questions included to test candidates' familiarity with well-known or characteristic side effects. In particular, candidates who have not yet spent a significant amount of time working in general practice will be using a different set of drugs in their day-to-day practice and so may not be as familiar with some drugs commonly used in general practice. Although there is not a definitive list to be memorized, below is a list of some side effects characteristically associated with certain drugs.

As training progresses and in preparation for this exam, make a note of any unusual side effects identified in day-to-day practice or while studying.

Characteristic drug side effects

- Altered colour vision – sildenafil
- Dry eyes – propranolol
- Double vision – carbamazepine
- Cataract – prednisolone
- Orange–red tears – rifampicin
- Photosensitivity – tetracycline antibiotics

- Nephrotoxicity – aminoglycoside antibiotics
- Peripheral neuropathy – tricyclic antidepressants
- Agranulocytosis/neutropenia – clozapine
- Gum hypertrophy – phenytoin
- Gynaecomastia – cimetidine
- Bronchoconstriction – beta-blockers
- Gastric upset – NSAIDs.

AKT Paper 6: Questions

1–6) *PV bleeding in pregnancy*
Match the diagnosis:

A Inevitable miscarriage
B Missed miscarriage
C Placental abruption
D Placenta praevia
E Threatened miscarriage
F Ectopic pregnancy

1) A 6/40 pregnant woman presents with PV spotting. On PV exam the os is closed.

2) An 8/40 pregnant female presents with PV bleeding. On PV exam the os is open.

3) A 14/40 pregnant female is noted to have a uterus that is small for dates. The os is closed.

4) A 22/40 pregnant female comes for an antenatal check. No fetal heart sounds are present.

5) A 29/40 pregnant female presents with severe lower abdominal pain and PV bleed.

6) An 8/40 pregnant woman presents with minimal PV bleeding, dizziness and right iliac fossa pain.

7–9) *Methotrexate*
For each of the following clinical scenarios, match the appropriate action:

A Continue current dose of methotrexate
B Decrease by 2.5 mg weekly
C Discontinue methotrexate
D Increase by 2.5 mg weekly

7) A 38-year-old woman is on methotrexate for rheumatoid arthritis. Her WCC is 8×10^9/L and platelets 220×10^9/L. 2 months later her WCC is 3×10^9/L and the platelets 100×10^9/L.

8) A 26-year-old man is on methotrexate for rheumatoid arthritis. He presents with a cough. On examination he is afebrile and the chest is clear. His WCC is 11×10^9/L and platelets 200×10^9/L.

9) A 50-year-old woman is on methotrexate for rheumatoid arthritis. She has been on it for 2 months but her symptoms are only mildly improving. She is still in considerable pain. The WCC is 12×10^9/L and the platelet count is 250×10^9/L.

10) *Factorial trials*
While updating your knowledge on recent advances in cancer care, you come across a factorial trial.
This is:

A A trial which takes more than one causative factor into account
B A trial in which patients are stratified into two or more groups
C A trial where each patient receives both the active drug and the placebo treatment
D A trial where more than one treatment is being tested simultaneously
E A trial where more than one treatment is tested sequentially

11) *95% confidence intervals*
A 95% confidence interval is one where:

A 95% of the data fall within the 95% confidence interval range
B there is a 95% chance that the true value falls within the confidence interval
C there is a 95% chance that the study value is correct
D there is a 95% chance that the two groups are not statistically significantly different
E there is a 95% chance that the finding is clinically significant

12) *Relative risk reduction*

A double-blind, placebo-controlled trial looked at a preventive treatment for influenza for patients in care homes. 5000 patients were randomized to receive treatment A or placebo. The patients were followed up for 1 year to determine if any of them developed influenza. 2.5% of the patients who received placebo developed influenza compared to 1.5% of the patients allocated to treatment A. **Which of the following statements is TRUE regarding the new treatment?**

A Treatment A produced a 1% proportional risk reduction in influenza
B The number needed to treat (NNT) to prevent influenza in
   1 patient = 100/1.5 = 67
C Treatment A produced a 1.5% absolute risk reduction in influenza
D Treatment A produced a 40% proportional risk reduction in influenza
E Treatment A produced a 40% absolute risk reduction in influenza

13) *Standard deviations*

In a study graph showing values in a normal distribution curve, what percentage of data lies within ± 1 standard deviation of the mean?

A 50%
B 68%
C 75%
D 88%
E 95%

14) *Case-control studies*

Which of the following is TRUE regarding case-control study design?

A It can only be used to look at a single possible risk factor for a disease in any one study
B It is a poor design choice for investigating rare diseases
C It is a good study design to investigate the cause of rare diseases
D It compares an outcome of interest in cases and controls
E It is a good study design to identify a rare cause of a disease

15) *Treatments for depression*

Each of the following is an evidence-based treatment for adults with depression EXCEPT:

A Cognitive behavioural therapy
B Selective serotonin reuptake inhibitors
C Interpersonal psychotherapy
D Lithium
E St John's wort

16) *Continuous and categorical data*
Regarding the description and comparison of two groups of data, which ONE of the following statements is true?

A Categorical data should be analysed using student's t test
B Skewed, continuous data should be summarized using median and range and compared using non-parametric statistical tests
C Skewed, continuous data should be summarized using mean and standard deviation and analysed using parametric statistical tests
D Normally distributed, continuous data should be summarized using mean and standard deviation and analysed using non-parametric statistical tests
E Normally distributed, continuous data should be summarized using median and standard deviation and analysed using non-parametric statistical tests

17) *Lower urinary tract symptoms in men*
For men suffering lower urinary tract symptoms due to enlarged prostate, the TWO first line drug therapy options are:

A 5α-reductase inhibitors
B Ipratropium bromide
C Benzatropine
D Alpha-blockers
E Saw palmetto

18) *Prostate-specific antigen testing*
A 65-year-old gentleman attends your clinic suffering from lower urinary tract symptoms (LUTS). He has an enlarged prostate. His MSSU is negative and he has no symptoms suggestive of a urinary tract infection. His PSA level is 4.4.
The level in men aged 60–69 above which urgent Urology referral is required is:

A ≥ 2.0 ng/mL
B ≥ 3.0 ng/mL
C ≥ 4.0 ng/mL
D ≥ 5.0 ng/mL
E ≥ 5.5 ng/mL

19) *Management of peripheral disease*

Your registrar is undertaking an audit of your care of patients who suffer from peripheral vascular disease.

The following steps should be taken in the management of peripheral artery disease in primary care EXCEPT:

A All patients should be on a statin to achieve a 25% reduction in cholesterol

B Consider ACE inhibitors in all patients, even if normotensive

C Prescribe aspirin 75 mg daily

D Prescribe cilostazol for the first 3–6 months as a first line therapy

E Screen for type II diabetes

20–25) *Asylum or refugee status*

For each of the following situations, select the most appropriate term:

A Asylum seeker

B Naturalization

C Investor status

D Family reunion

E Refugee status

F Refusal

G Definite leave to remain

20) The wife and two children of a man who has been successful in his application for asylum.

21) A 45-year-old Chinese man who fled persecution has been living in the UK legally for 5 years. He would now like to apply for British citizenship.

22) A 55-year-old Iraqi woman has submitted an application for protection under the 1951 Geneva Convention and is waiting for her claim to be settled by the Home Office.

23) A 35-year-old man from the Democratic Republic of Congo has been granted Indefinite Leave to Remain by the Home Office due to the torture he suffered for his political beliefs. He has been in the UK for 1 year.

24) A 29-year-old man from Afghanistan is living legally in the UK. His application to the Home Office did not strictly meet the requirements for refugee status but he was allowed to remain in the UK for the next 5 years. He is expected to return to his home country if the situation improves.

25) A 57-year-old multimillionaire businessman wishes to live and work in the UK. He has not suffered persecution but is fearful that war in his home country has destabilized the economy and he wishes to start a UK-based business as soon at possible.

26–29) *Hand pain*

For each of the following clinical scenarios, select the most likely diagnosis:

A Carpal tunnel syndrome
B De Quervain's disease
C Dupuytren's contracture
D Scaphoid fracture
E Trigger thumb
F Repetitive strain injury
G Sprain

26) A 40-year-old woman presents with a swollen left wrist. She works as a hotel maid. On examination there is swelling over the styloid process of the radius with pain on forced flexion and adduction of the thumb.

27) A 45-year-old woman works as a hospital administrator. She complains of hand pain. On further questioning her pain is limited to the first 3½ digits of her right hand. She has no thenar wasting but suffers occasional pins and needles. Her pain is worse at night when she has to get up and shake her hands.

28) A 45-year-old woman works as a hospital administrator. She complains of hand pain. Her pain does not affect her fingers, but manifests as wrist pain which radiates proximally up her arms. Her pain is worse at night but improves at the weekend.

29) A 23-year-old man had been in a fight 2 weeks ago when he sustained punch injuries and fell onto both hands. His left hand had been painful but Accident and Emergency X-rays at the time had shown no fracture. He presents to your surgery because he is still having pain in his left thumb. On examination, the only tenderness he has occurs on compression of his anatomical snuff box.

30–35) *Eye conditions*
For each of the following clinical scenarios, choose the most likely diagnosis:

A Acute conjunctivitis
B Acute iritis
C Central retinal artery occlusion
D Central retinal vein occlusion
E Closed angled glaucoma
F Posterior communicating aneurysm
G Retinal detachment
H Vitreous haemorrhage

30) An 8-year-old child presents with sudden diplopia, ptosis and a lateral diverging eye.

31) A 60-year-old woman complains of a 'curtain coming down' over her right eye with painless loss of vision. She mentions seeing flashing lights first.

32) A 40-year-old man complains of a painful red eye with photophobia and pain on accommodation. The pupil is irregular.

33) A 70-year-old woman presents with a cloudy cornea, reduced visual acuity and painful red eye.

34) A 75-year-old woman presents with sudden loss of vision in the left eye with acuity reduced to finger counting. The fundus resembles a 'bloodstorm'.

35) A 60-year-old woman presents with sudden loss of vision in the right eye with acuity reduced to light perception. The retina appears white with a cherry-red spot on the macula. She comments that she had transient blindness before full blindness of the right eye.

36) *Osteoporosis*
A 60-year-old woman sustains a hip fracture. Upon discharge from hospital, you decide to put her on medication for osteoporosis.
Besides Calcichew-D3 Forte, you should add which SINGLE medication:

A Alendronic acid
B Calcitonin
C Raloxifene
D HRT
E Tiludronic acid

37) *Allergy testing*
A 15-year-old boy attends the surgery worried about his family history of peanut allergy. He had a cousin who died from a peanut allergy. He avoids peanuts in his diet and has never reacted himself. He has a history of eczema and asthma, which have always been well controlled.
Which of the following options is the most useful initial test?

A Nasal smear
B Patch test
C Serum CRP
D Serum allergen-specific IgE test
E Skin prick test

38–42) *Haematological conditions*
For each of the patients select the most likely diagnosis:

A Acute lymphoblastic leukaemia
B Acute myeloid leukaemia
C Chronic granulocytic leukaemia
D Chronic lymphocytic leukaemia
E Non-Hodgkin's lymphoma
F Hodgkin's lymphoma
G Iron-deficiency anaemia
H Multiple myeloma
I Sickle-cell anaemia

38) A 14-year-old male presents with recurrent gum bleeding, sore throat, mouth ulcers and malaise. On examination he has a palpable spleen. Blood tests show elevated WCC with decreased platelets. Blood film shows a few blast cells. His father works in a gas station with regular exposure to petrol.

39) A 25-year-old woman presents with an enlarged, painless cervical lymph node. She also reports drenching night sweats and has lost weight. Peripheral blood smear shows Reed–Sternberg cells with a bilobed, mirror-imaged nucleus.

40) A 70-year-old man presents with recurrent chest infections and chronic back pain. Blood tests reveal anaemia and elevated urea and creatinine. Blood tests reveal an elevated ESR and calcium. Bone marrow reveals an abundance of malignant plasma cells.

41) An 8-year-old boy presents with swelling of the hands and feet. Hb is 8 mg/dL. Peripheral blood smear reveals target cells and elongated crescent-shaped red blood cells.

42) A 65-year-old woman presents with dysphagia. She is also noted to have spoon-shaped fingernails and a smooth tongue. Blood smear reveals microcytic, hypochromic blood cells.

43–46) *Urinary incontinence*
For each of the following patients, select the most likely diagnosis:

A Cystocoele
B Disc prolapse
C Multiple sclerosis
D Pelvic floor prolapse
E Senile vaginitis
F Urinary tract infection
G Vesico-vaginal fistula

43) A 55-year-old woman reports persistent dribbling urinary incontinence following her vaginal hysterectomy. It occurs on movement but has not been improved by pelvic floor exercises. She does not have urinary urgency or any feeling of prolapse.

44) A 60-year-old man presents with back pain. On examination, he has saddle anaesthesia, urinary incontinence and loss of anal tone.

45) A 70-year-old woman reports 3 months of urinary incontinence. She is ashamed to bring this up with you. Coughing makes matters worse. MSU is normal.

46) A 40-year-old woman presents with double vision, weakness in both legs and urinary incontinence.

47) *Caldicott principles of confidentiality*
Your practice manager has asked you to review the practice policy on use of patient information.
Which of the following is NOT a correct interpretation of the Caldicott Report regarding confidentiality?

A Access to personally identifiable information should be on a strict need-to-know basis
B Consent should be sought to use anonymous patient information
C Justify the purpose of information use
D Understand and comply with the law
E Do not use personally identifiable information unless it is absolutely necessary
F Everyone should be aware of his or her responsibilities

48) *Assessment of risk in body fluid contacts*
When assessing the risk of a bodily fluid contact, which of the following is considered to be the HIGHEST risk?

A Exposure of intact skin to known HIV-positive blood
B A patient in the GP out-of-hours service vomits blood over the waiting room chairs
C Exposure of a cut to blood known to be positive for hepatitis C.
D Exposure of a cut on the hand to blood from a patient in general practice
E Exposure of a cut on the hand to known hepatitis B-positive blood. The nurse has been adequately immunized against hepatitis B

49) *Brief intervention models*

You wish to encourage smoking cessation in your practice. You decide to employ the FRAMES brief intervention model.

Which of the following is NOT part of this model?

A Firm – a firm approach from the healthcare professional is more likely to gain a positive result

B Responsibility – emphasis that the harmful behaviour is by choice

C Advice – explicit advice on changing the harmful behaviour

D Menu – offering alternative goals and strategies

E Empathy – the role of the counsellor is important

F Self-efficacy – instilling optimism that the chosen goals can be achieved

50) *Screening tools*

You wish to identify patients in your practice who might have an alcohol problem using a screening questionnaire.

Which of the following is NOT a screening questionnaire to identify possible alcohol problems?

A CAGE questionnaire

B MAST questionnaire

C SCOFF questionnaire

D AUDIT questionnaire

E SADQ questionnaire

51–53) *Abdominal swelling*

For the following scenarios, select the most likely diagnosis:

A Alcoholic liver disease

B Pregnancy

C Irritable bowel syndrome

D Fibroid disease

E Uterine carcinoma

F Colorectal carcinoma

51) A 42-year-old lady presents with abdominal swelling associated with constipation and nausea. Her periods have been irregular for the past year but absent for the past 2 months. Her appetite is unchanged. She drinks a glass of wine per night. She has not noticed any change in her weight.

52) A 42-year-old man presents with abdominal swelling. He has not noticed any change in his weight but cannot now do up his trousers. He refuses to be pinned down on how much he drinks. He admits he drinks every day but denies he has a problem.

53) A 45-year-old woman presents with abdominal pain and swelling associated with constipation. Her periods are regular and no more heavy than usual. She drinks only occasionally. There has been no change in her weight. Her pain is relieved on passing a bowel movement. Between episodes of constipation, she suffers from occasional diarrhoea. She has no blood in her bowel movements but does have mucus occasionally.

54) *Referrals for men with lower urinary tract symptoms*
A man complains of poor urine flow and having to get up through the night to urinate.
Which of the following would NOT require urgent referral?

A An elevated age-specific PSA in an otherwise well 50-year-old man
B A 60-year-old man with a hard irregular prostate swelling
C Painful macroscopic haematuria in an adult
D A 51-year-old man with a palpable renal mass
E A 55-year-old man with longstanding lower urinary tract symptoms whose U&Es show evidence of chronic renal failure

55–59) *ENT conditions*
For each of the following patients, identify the most likely diagnosis:

A Acoustic neuroma
B Herpes zoster oticus
C Ménière's disease
D Occupational noise damage
E Otosclerosis
F Presbyacusis

55) A 35-year-old pregnant woman presents with bilateral conductive hearing loss. Both tympanic membranes appear normal.

56) A 70-year-old man presents with gradual onset of bilateral sensorineural hearing loss.

57) A 65-year-old woman presents with sudden onset of unilateral facial weakness and sensorineural hearing loss. She is also noted to have vesicles in the external auditory meatus.

58) A 50-year-old woman presents with unilateral low-frequency sensorineural hearing loss and vertigo.

59) A 50-year-old man presents with a gradual onset of unilateral sensorineural hearing loss and unilateral tinnitus.

60) *Cervical screening*

You are a GP in central London. A 21-year-old woman is concerned about her risk of cervical cancer as she has been sexually active since the age of 14. She comments that she has never been called for a cervical smear.

What is the age range of cervical screening in England?

A 18–65
B 20–64
C 25–49
D 25–64
E 20–70

61) *Breast screening*

A 50-year-old woman with no family history attends requesting mammography to screen for breast cancer. She has no lumps or symptoms to report.

What age range for breast cancer screening with mammography is recommended for women between the ages of:

A 40–60
B 45–60
C 45–65
D 50–64
E 50–70

62) *Human papilloma virus vaccination*

The father of a 15-year-old girl attends your surgery to ask about the possibility of having her vaccinated against cervical cancer. He is not aware of her being sexually active yet but is keen to have her vaccinated early.

At what age is the human papilloma virus vaccine routinely given?

A 10–11
B 12–13
C 14–15
D 15–16
E 16–17

63) *Faith considerations*
Below is a list of considerations which may apply regarding healthcare. To which of the below World Faiths might these apply?

- Patients may not cut their hair. If hair is required to be removed (e.g. prior to an operation), they may wish to have it returned to them for disposal.
- Family may expect to be involved in the decision-making processes relating to the diagnosis and treatment of their relatives, and will also expect to be able to care for their relatives in hospital.
- Human life is considered to be sacrosanct and begins at the moment of conception. Followers may not be comfortable using forms of contraception, which act by preventing implantation.

A Buddhism
B Hinduism
C Islam
D Judaism
E Sikhism

64) *The Sicily statement on evidence–based practice*
You are writing a statement for your practice based on the Sicily statement on evidence-based practice.
Which of the following is NOT part of this statement?

A Practice based on personal experience
B Systemic retrieval of best evidence available
C Critical appraisal of evidence for validity, clinical relevance and applicability
D Application of results in practice
E Evaluation of performance

65) *Anaphylaxis*
A 45-year-old gentleman collapses in the waiting room with symptoms suggestive of an anaphylactic reaction. He has a history of severe peanut allergy.
What is the appropriate dose of intramuscular injection of adrenaline (epinephrine) for anaphylactic shock?

A 0.15 mL 1 in 1000 adrenaline
B 0.5 mL 1 in 1000 adrenaline
C 0.5 mL 1 in 10 000 adrenaline
D 1 mL 1 in 1000 adrenaline
E 1 mL 1 in 10 000 adrenaline

66–71) *Alcohol units*
For the drinks below estimate the number of alcohol units:

A 1 unit
B 2 units
C 3 units
D 4 units
E 5 units
F 6 units
G 10 units
H 20 units
I 30 units
J 40 units

66) A large glass (250 mL) of white wine 12% ABV.

67) A standard glass (50 mL) of sherry 20% ABV.

68) A 500 ml bottle of 8% ABV German beer.

69) A half litre bottle of 40% ABV whisky.

70) A 750 mL bottle of 80 proof vodka brought from Russia by a friend.

71) A single, standard measure of whisky.

72–76) *Evidence–based Management of lower back pain*
For each of the clinical cases below select the SINGLE best management option:

A Advise bedrest and NSAIDs
B Arrange urgent referral
C Assess for yellow flags
D Continue normal daily activities and prescribe paracetamol
E Emergency referral
F Specialist referral if no better in 6 weeks after conservative management

72) A 50-year-old man presents with back pain. He has lumbosacral pain with no neurological symptoms and no radiating features.

73) A 56-year-old man presents with 2 months of thoracic back pain and weight loss. On examination he has structural deformity and widespread neurological symptoms.

74) A 30-year-old woman presents with buttock pain radiating down to her toes. Straight leg raise reproduces the pain.

75) A 60-year-old man presents with urinary inconti anaesthesia and severe back pain. He had felt fit and this.

76) A 40-year-old man requests repeated Med3 certificates fo pain. He initially hurt his back while lifting boxes for a f was moving house.

77) *Funnel plots*
Which of the following is TRUE regarding the use of funnel p meta-analysis?

A An asymmetrical funnel plot suggests there may be publication
B A symmetrical funnel plot suggests there is no benefit in the drug being studied
C It is inappropriate to include a funnel plot when carrying out a meta-analysis
D An asymmetrical funnel plot means no conclusions can be drawn from the data
E A symmetrical funnel plot suggests that the studies used were underpowered

78–80) *Gynaecological cancers*
Match the following gynaecological cancers with the MOST likely age groups at risk:

A Uterine carcinoma
B Ovarian carcinoma
C Cervical carcinoma
D Vulval carcinoma

78) Age group 20–64 with a median age of 52 years.

79) Over 40 with a median age of 60 years.

80) Majority occurs in the 65–70 year-old age group.

81) *Coeliac disease*
A 7-year-old boy presents with recurrent abdominal bloating, weight loss and diarrhoea. He is in the 5th percentile for height and weight.
Which screening investigation is the SINGLE most sensitive?

A Endomysial antibodies
B Faecal fat estimation
C Full blood count
D Urea and electrolytes
E Vitamin B12/folate levels

82–92) *Modes of inheritance*
Match the following genetic conditions with their mode of inheritance:

A Autosomal dominant
B Autosomal recessive
C X-linked recessive
D X-linked dominant
E Polygenic inheritance

82) Achondroplasia

83) Adult polycystic kidney disease

84) Becker muscular dystrophy

85) Club foot

86) Haemochromatosis

87) Marfan's syndrome

88) Neural tube defects

89) Red–green colour blindness

90) Sickle-cell anaemia

91) Vitamin D-resistant rickets

92) Type I diabetes

93–95) *Cancer mortality*
Put the following cancers in order of the increasing causes of cancer mortality:

A Breast carcinoma
B Colorectal carcinoma
C Lung carcinoma
D Melanoma carcinoma
E Prostate carcinoma

93) Commonest cause of cancer death in males and females

94) Second most common cause of death in males and females

95) Third most common cause of death in males and females

96) *Cancer mortality*
Which is the SECOND most common cause of cancer mortality in men?

A Colorectal carcinoma
B Gastric carcinoma
C Lung carcinoma
D Oesophageal carcinoma
E Prostate carcinoma

97) *Cancer mortality*
Which is the SECOND most common cause of cancer mortality in women?

A Breast carcinoma
B Colorectal carcinoma
C Lung carcinoma
D Other carcinomas
E Ovarian carcinoma

98) *Domestic abuse*
A woman attends your surgery with bruising on her face. You suspect domestic violence to be the cause.
Which of the following puts her at higher risk of becoming a victim of domestic violence?

A Age over 30
B Asian ethnicity
C Did not complete high school education
D Unplanned pregnancy
E White ethnicity

99) *Domestic abuse*
A woman attends your surgery with bruising on her face. You suspect domestic violence to be the cause.
Which of the following makes it more likely that a person would choose violent behaviour toward a partner?

A Being in a same sex relationship
B History of alcoholism
C Outgoing personality
D Being in a manual job
E Poor literacy levels

100) *Gynaecomastia*
In the following scenarios, all patients are 50-year-old men with a 2-month history of gynaecomastia.
Which of the following additional symptoms are LEAST likely to be associated with a sinister diagnosis?

A 2-month history of daily headache
B 2 months of unexplained severe lethargy
C 1-year history of cardiac failure with atrial fibrillation
D Currently being investigated for a testicular lump
E A man with a strong family history of female breast cancer

1) E Threatened miscarriage
PV bleeding is very common in early pregnancy. Bleeding itself defines threatened miscarriage. It causes a lot of anxiety though most are associated with ongoing pregnancy.

2) A Inevitable miscarriage
An open os defines inevitable miscarriage. Around 30% of pregnancies will end in spontaneous abortion. Some will need surgical intervention to remove retained products of conception, but most will complete spontaneously. Monitor for temperature as evidence of sepsis.

3) B Missed miscarriage
Termed missed miscarriage due to fetal death. It may be some time before the patient starts to bleed. 8/10 miscarriages occur within the first 12 weeks of pregnancy.

4) B Missed miscarriage
Without a dating scan prior to passing of the products, it is impossible to say at what gestation there was a loss of fetal heartbeat.

5) C Placental abruption
This is premature detachment of the placenta from the uterus. It is an obstetric emergency. Posterior detachment may manifest as back pain. A small abruption may require monitoring only. A larger abruption will require immediate delivery of the child. Note that PV bleeding may not occur, particularly in a fundal abruption.

6) F Ectopic pregnancy
Unilateral abdominal pain and vaginal bleeding with previous amenorrhoea is an ectopic pregnancy until proven otherwise.

7) C Discontinue methotrexate
Medication errors have occurred with methotrexate, mostly due to its weekly dosing. Methotrexate must be stopped if any profound drop in WCC or platelets occurs. Patients should be carefully advised of the dose and frequency. Only one strength of tablet should be prescribed and dispensed. In addition, 5 mg folate should be given the day after each dose of methotrexate.

8) A Continue current dose of methotrexate

The patient is warned to report immediately the onset of any of the following:

- Sore throat, bruising and mouth ulcers (blood disorders)
- Nausea, vomiting, abdominal discomfort and dark urine (liver toxicity)
- Shortness of breath (respiratory disorders)

9) D Increase by 2.5 mg weekly

Methotrexate dosing, as with all immunosuppressants, is a matter of balancing symptom control with limiting side effects. Monitoring should include FBC, LFTs and U&Es weekly until therapy stabilizes, then 2–3 monthly. Methotrexate is usually managed via a shared care protocol between primary and secondary care.

10) D A trial where more than one treatment is being tested simultaneously

Most trials evaluate just one treatment. A factorial trial evaluates more than one treatment simultaneously. For example, in the ISIS-2 study, a comparison was made between placebo and each of two drugs: streptokinase and aspirin. Myocardial infarction patients were randomized to receive IV streptokinase alone, aspirin alone, both active drugs, or double placebo. The trial showed that each of the drugs produced about a 25% reduction in mortality, also that their effects were additive. These trials may still be adequately blinded with placebo use, but require more subjects to achieve appropriate power.

11) B There is a 95% chance that the true value falls within the confidence interval

The 95% confidence interval (95% CI) is a statistical measure of how close a study mean is likely to be to the real value. It is the range around a study value where there is a 95% chance that the true value lies. Remember that statistical and clinical significance are not the same. A very large study can have very narrow 95% CIs (or very small p values) for very small differences, which may be of no clinical significance at all. A small study, however, may fail to show a statistically significant effect even if the effect is both large and clinically important.

12) D Treatment A produced a 40% proportional risk reduction in influenza

Proportional risk reduction is another term for relative risk reduction. Treatment A reduces the risk of influenza from 2.5% to 1.5%. This is:

- absolute risk reduction of 2.5 to 1.5 = 1%
- relative risk reduction of 1/2.5 = 40%
- number needed to treat = 1/absolute risk reduction = 1/0.01 = 100.

13) B 68%

Standard deviation is a measure of the spread of values around a mean. In a tall, thin graph, the standard deviation will be small; in a short, broad graph, the standard deviation will be much larger. Each graph might have the same mean.

- approximately 68% of the values lie within ± 1 SD of the mean
- approximately 95% of the values lie within ± 2 SDs of the mean
- approximately 99.7% of the values lie within ± 3 SDs of the mean
- *exactly* 95% of the values lie within ± 1.96 standard deviations of the mean (hence 2.5% lie in each tail).

14) C It is a good study design to investigate the cause of rare diseases
Case-control studies are retrospective studies taking a group of cases with an outcome (or disease) of interest and matching them to a group of controls. The groups are then compared for exposures of interest (or causes). This is the opposite to cohort studies, which are prospective and used to look at outcomes of interest. Case-control studies are good for investigating rare diseases and can be used to identify multiple possible exposure risk factors.

15) D Lithium
Evidence-based treatments for depression include ECT, especially for severe depression. In mild to moderate depression there is no real difference in efficacy between different classes of antidepressant; however, there are big differences in side effects. Be aware that tricyclics and SSRIs might make suicidal ideation worse on initial treatment. Exercise is useful in mild–moderate depression.

Lithium and pindolol, a beta-blocker, are sometimes used in treatment-resistant depression to augment the effects of antidepressants; however, there is not yet any conclusive evidence that they are efficacious.

Continuing antidepressants following recovery can reduce the risk of relapse.

16) B Skewed, continuous data should be summarized using median and range and compared using non-parametric statistical tests
Categorical variables are not continuous; for example, dead versus alive or event versus no event occurring. Categorical data can be examined using the chi-squared test. Normally distributed continuous data is, for example, blood pressure or blood sugar measurements. They should be summarized by stating the mean and standard deviation and analysed using parametric statistical tests (for example student's t-test). Skewed continuous data, i.e. data that are not normally distributed, should be summarized by stating the median and range. They should by analysed using non-parametric statistical tests (such as analysis of variance).

17) D Alpha-blockers
A 5α-reductase inhibitors
Men with uncomplicated lower urinary tract symptoms arising from benign enlargement of the prostate should reduce fluid intake in the evening and avoid caffeine initially.

If troublesome symptoms persist, alpha-blockers (e.g. doxazocin) should be offered for 2–4 weeks. If the patient cannot tolerate the side effects or the prostate is estimated to be greater than 40 mL, 5α-reductase inhibitors (e.g. finasteride) should be offered. Evidence-based medicine has shown that saw palmetto (*Serenoa repens*), a herbal supplement, improved overall self-rated urinary symptoms from baseline compared with placebo but long-term safety has not been addressed. Men with visible haematuria, dysuria, renal failure or urinary retention should be offered referral for specialist assessment under the 2-week wait scheme.

18) C ≥4.0 ng/mL
The PSA levels above which urgent Urology referral is required are as follows:

Age (years)	Refer to Urology if PSA (ng/mL) is
50–59	≥3.0
60–69	≥4.0
4.0≥70	≥5.0

A question in the AKT would be unlikely to involve precise memorization of PSA levels such as this; however, an EMQ might involve a number of clinical cases of men with LUTS symptoms while asking you to decide if the cases need referral at all, routinely or urgently.

19) D Prescribe cilostazol for the first 3–6 months as a first line therapy
Cilostazol is a useful adjunct in patients who have unacceptable symptoms despite 3–6 months of best medical treatment and has been shown to increase walking distance in patients with claudication. Peripheral vascular disease should be managed as aggressively as angina as a marker of risk of a cardiovascular event and sudden death. This should include all of the medical treatments that would ordinarily be considered to reduce cardiovascular risk: antiplatelet agents, antihypertensives and cholesterol-lowering agents.
    ACE inhibitor therapy is an important consideration but be aware of the possibility of undiagnosed renovascular disease and start with caution.

20) D Family reunion
One spouse and children of that marriage under the age of 18 are granted the same leave to remain as their family member.

21) B Naturalization
Naturalization is the process by which British citizenship is obtained by non-British adults. British naturalization is also known as British citizenship. As a British citizen you have the right to live in the UK

permanently and are free to leave and re-enter the UK without restriction. Must have lived legally in the UK for 5 years and held indefinite leave to remain official recognition for 1 year at the time of application.

22) A Asylum seeker

An asylum seeker (person seeking refugee status) is a person who has submitted an application for protection under the 1951 Geneva Convention and is waiting for their claim to be settled by the Home Office. A person is not termed a refugee until their application has been granted by the Home Office.

23) E Rufugee status

Refugee status is given when the Home Office considers that the person fits into the definition as set out by the 1951 UN Convention Relating to Refugees. According to this definition, a refugee is a person who:
- has a well-founded fear of persecution for reasons of race, religion, nationality, membership of a particular social group or political opinion
- is outside the country they belong to or normally reside in
- is unable or unwilling to return home for fear of persecution.

May be with or without indefinite leave to remain. Refugees do not automatically qualify for indefinite leave to remain but more commonly will be given a definite 5 years to remain initially.

24) G Definate leave to stay

Indefinite Leave to Remain (ILR) is settlement in the UK. There are no conditions attached to it and someone with ILR can always work. After a certain period, those with settlement can apply for British citizenship. Usually associated with refugee status but those who do not strictly fit the definition of the 1951 UN Convention may be given the discretionary right to stay for a specific period on humanitarian grounds. This is known as Humanitarian Protection or Discretionary Leave.

25) C Investor status

Investor status is granted to those able to invest a large amount of money into UK businesses. The work permit only allows the holder to work in self-employment.

26) B De Quervain's disease

Tenosynovitis causes pain and stiffness in the line of the tendon and crepitus over the affected tendon. It can occur in any tendon but most commonly in the thumb as described above. Pain on forced flexion and adduction of the thumb is a positive Finkelstein's sign for De Quervain's tenosynovitis (stenosing tenovaginitis). The cause of the condition is unknown; however, wringing motions of the hands, e.g. drying out clothes, aggravate the condition. Treatment may involve steroid injection around the tendons or surgical decompression.

27) A Carpal tunnel syndrome
Carpal tunnel syndrome is a chronic compression of the median nerve with pain, numbness and thenar wasting. Worse at night, it can be managed by using night splints, steroid injections or surgery in severe cases. Diuretics may be helpful. If obesity is a causative factor, losing weight can help. Physical examination could include:
- Phalen's test, where hyperflexion of the wrist for 1 minute triggers the symptoms
- Tinel's test, where tapping over the carpal tunnel causes symptoms.

28) F Repetitive strain injury
Repetitive strain injury causes wrist and arm pain. Symptoms vary depending on the movement involved. Most commonly related to work or computer games. There are no physical signs. Treatment is with physiotherapy and cessation of the causative activity.

29) D Scaphoid fracture
Scaphoid fracture occurs following a fall onto the hand. It does not always show up on initial X-ray. If clinically suspected by tenderness over the anatomical snuffbox, patients should have a cast and have the wrist re-X-rayed 2 weeks later. It is an important diagnosis to make because of the potential complications of avascular necrosis and non-union.

30) F Posterior communicating aneurysm
This child has an oculomotor (CN III) palsy where the eye looks 'down and out'. Other signs include proptosis, pain and fixed pupil dilatation. The likely cause here is a congenital berry aneurysm on the posterior communicating artery on the circle of Willis. Other causes include cavernous sinus lesions, tumour and diabetes.

31) G Retinal detachment
In retinal detachment the outer retinal pigment epithelium separates from the inner neuro-retina. Risk factors include severe myopia (due to elongated eye shape), congenital cataract and following cataract surgery. It is essential to identify early signs which may allow surgery to potentially stop progression and preserve sight, in particular to preserve the macula. Early symptoms include flashes and floaters: flashes are due to abnormal retinal stimulation; floaters are due to vitreous haemorrhage. Patients complain of a shadow or curtain coming down over their vision. Any sudden loss of vision should be referred as an emergency.

32) B Acute iritis
Acute iritis (or anterior uveitis) presents with pain, photophobia, redness and watery eye. Examination shows circumcorneal redness and a small, possibly irregular pupil. A hypopyon may be present. This presents as a fluid level seen in the cornea and is anterior chamber pus. Causes include Behçet's disease and ankylosing spondylitis. Treatment is with steroid drops and mydriatics to dilate the pupil.

33) E Closed angled glucoma

Closed angled glaucoma classically presents with painful visual loss with 'haloes around lights'. In this way it differs from retinal detachment. Can be brought on by dilatation of pupils at night or by dilatation of pupils by mydriatics. The cloudy cornea is due to oedema. Pupil is fixed and dilated due to raised intraocular pressure. It may be oval. There may be circumcorneal redness and the eyeball will feel hard due to raised intraocular pressure.

34) D Central retinal vein occlusion

A sudden, painful loss of vision in one eye occurs in central retinal vein occlusion. An occlusion in a branch would result in partial visual loss. The 'bloodstorm' appearance is due to engorged retinal veins and oedema, leading to retinal haemorrhage. Causes include chronic glaucoma, which causes increased pressure, which occludes the central retinal vein. Other causes include conditions which cause increased blood viscosity such as arteriosclerosis, polycythaemia and hyperlipidaemia.

35) C Central retinal artery occlusion

Unlike central retinal vein occlusion, central retinal artery occlusion is painless. A relative afferent pupillary defect is present (Marcus–Gunn pupil), i.e. the affected pupil reacts poorly to light where the consensual light reaction is normal. Test this by using the 'swing test'. The retina is pale due to oedema with a 'cherry red spot' at the macula. Optic atrophy occurs without treatment. Occlusion occurs due to either vasospasm or emboli. Embolic disease may present with a 'flickering' in the vision as tiny emboli briefly interrupt blood flow before disintegrating and passing through. Sudden visual loss then occurs when a larger embolus occurs. Risk factors are the same as for other forms of cardiovascular disease: diabetes, smoking and hypertension.

36) A Alendronic acid

Both alendronate and risedronate (both bisphosphonates) are once-weekly preparations, which is more amenable for patients who dislike daily tablets. The classic dowager's hump is pathognomonic for severe osteoporosis without imaging. A lateral back X-ray should be obtained if osteoporosis is suspected and confirmed by DEXA scan. A value ≥ 2.5 standard deviations below the young adult female value is the WHO definition for osteoporosis. It is mandatory to put your patient on osteoporosis prophylaxis if you prescribe long-term corticosteroids. Recent evidence shows that repeated short courses of steroids may be more detrimental than long-term regular steroids! HRT is no longer recommended as prophylaxis against osteoporosis and should only be prescribed for 2–3 years maximum for relief of troublesome menopausal symptoms.

37) D Serum allergen-specific IgE test

RAST and ELISA are the laboratory techniques to measure serum-specific IgE. Skin prick testing is used to identify sensitivity to common allergens in atopy as an alternative to serum testing, but this is usually carried out in secondary care and so is not the correct answer here. Elevated serum CRP is a non-specific marker of inflammation and is of no diagnostic value in this context. A nasal cytological smear can be examined microscopically for eosinophilia to identify allergic rhinitis. As this is largely a clinical diagnosis, this test is not widely carried out. Patch testing is more useful to test for contact allergies than food allergies. Allergen-impregnated discs are placed on the skin, then the diameter of any erythematous reaction measured.

38) A Accute lymphoblastic leukaemia

This is an older than average acute lymphoblastic leukaemia (ALL) patient, with the usual range up to 10 years, with an additional peak in the fifth decade. Presenting symptoms match the consequences of bone marrow failure:

- anaemia causes pallor, lethargy, shortness of breath
- neutropenia causes infection, particularly of mouth and skin
- thrombocytopenia causes bruising and bleeding
- additional symptoms that can arise from organ infiltration include bone pain, lymphadenopathy, hepatosplenomegaly, testicular enlargement, and shortness of breath due to mediastinal lymphadenopathy.

ALL is the most common childhood leukaemia. It is a cancer of the lymphoid progenitor cells which can be detected in a peripheral blood smear. Prognosis is much poorer in older children and worse again in adults.

Note: Acute myeloid leukaemia (AML) presents in the same fashion due to bone marrow failure but tends to occur in a different age group. The median presentation age in AML is 60. It is the most common leukaemia of adulthood. Previous chemotherapy and radiotherapy are risk factors.

39) F Hodgkin's lymphoma

Lymphoma (neoplasia of lymphoid tissue) is divided into Hodgkin's (HL) and non-Hodgkin's lymphoma (NHL). It occurs mainly in lymph nodes and lymphoid organs and therefore usually cannot be diagnosed on peripheral blood film, unlike leukaemia. Some lymphomas can, however, be seen in the peripheral blood, although the presence of Reed–Sternberg cells in the peripheral blood is admittedly rare. NHL classification is complex and can be broken down into many subcategories (diffuse large B cell, Burkitt's, etc.), but for general practice purposes, the differences between HL and NHL are most important. Both present similarly with painless lymphadenopathy, night sweats, splenomegaly, weight loss and fevers.

	Hodgkin's lymphoma	Non-Hodgkin's lymphoma
Age at presentation	Bimodal: 15–35 then 50–70	Median 50
Spread	Contiguous, lymph node to lymph node, usually starting in the neck	Random throughout lymph nodes and organs
Histology	Polymorphic, with diagnostic Reed–Sternberg cells and many reactive cells	Monomorphic, predominantly malignant cells
Prognosis	Up to 80% 5-year survival	Varies depending on histology but in general much poorer than for HL

40) H Multiple myeloma
A B lymphocyte neoplasia growing mainly within bone marrow, causing infiltration, localized tumours and bone erosion. Presents with bone pain, chest infection, anaemia and renal failure. Diagnose by urinary Bence-Jones proteins or serum electrophoresis initially and bone marrow biopsy. Occurs generally in over 50s. Main sites are skull, vertebrae, ribs, pelvis and proximal long bones.

41) I Sickle-cell anaemia
MCQs will often point toward this diagnosis by stating the patient to be African, Mediterranean, Middle Eastern or Indian. Here, it is the description of the red blood cells. The swelling of the hands is a manifestation of the hand–foot syndrome, caused by chronic microinfarction in the small long bones of the hands and feet. It is associated with osteonecrosis, induration, swelling and erythema.

    In sickle cell trait, patients have <40% haemoglobin S. They have no symptoms unless hypoxic. In sickle cell anaemia, patients will be anaemic with a high reticulocyte count. Symptoms occur in 'sickling crises' acutely due to infarction. Patients tend to present with fever and pain.

42) G Iron-deficiency anaemia
Spoon-shaped fingernails (koilonychia) are a classic sign of iron deficiency anaemia. Smooth tongue or glossitis can be due to nutritional deficiency (iron, B12, folate, riboflavin or nicotinic acid) or idiopathic. Iron deficiency anaemia does not define an underlying cause. An underlying upper GI malignancy is implied here.

43) G Vesico-vaginal fistula

When assessing patients following surgery, establish if symptoms are likely to be part of normal recovery or surgical complication. Urinary tract infection following surgery would be another common cause of postoperative incontinence. Fistula formation is a risk following gynaecological or lower GI surgery.

44) B Disc prolapse

Red flags of back pain is a common MCQ

Back pain red flag signs

Age <20 or >55 years	Taking steroids
Non-mechanical back pain	Unwell
Thoracic pain	Weight loss
Past history of carcinoma	Widespread neurology
HIV	Structural deformity

45) D Pelvic Floor prolapse

Urinary incontinence remains a much more common problem in the population than ever presents to general practice. Although symptoms are traditionally split into stress and urge incontinence, in reality most patients have a mixed picture. Stress incontinence is treated with physiotherapy and surgery. Urge incontinence is treated by reducing caffeine intake, bladder training and antimuscarinic drugs. Pelvic floor prolapse can by treated using a vaginal ring pessary or surgery. Postmenopausal urinary incontinence may benefit from topical oestrogen therapy.

46) C Multiple sclerosis

If multiple sclerosis is suspected, refer to Neurology for confirmation of the diagnosis and specialist support. Bladder problems present in the form of urgency, frequency or incontinence. Think of this diagnosis in young people with multiple non-specific symptoms and fatigue; depression may initially predominate. Optic neuritis or other visual disturbance is the most common specific presenting complaint in multiple sclerosis.

47) B Consent should be sought to use anonymous patient information

The Caldicott Report set out a number of general principles that health and social care organizations should use when reviewing their use of client information and these are set out below:

1. Justify the purpose.
2. Do not use personally identifiable information unless it is absolutely necessary. This should not be used unless there is no alternative.
3. Use the minimum personally identifiable information. This should only be used where the use of such information is considered to be essential.

4. Access to personally identifiable information should be on a strictly need-to-know basis.
5. Everyone should be aware of their responsibilities. Action should be taken to ensure that those handling personally identifiable information are aware of their responsibilities and obligations to respect patient/client confidentiality.
6. Understand and comply with the law. There is no need to seek consent for completely anonymous information.

48) C Exposure of a cut to blood known to be positive for hepatitis C. When carrying out risk assessment, consider the mode of the injury and the risk factors in both involved parties. If the 'source' patient is available, it may be appropriate to obtain relevant history and blood samples to be tested urgently for blood-borne viruses.

Low risk exposures

- exposure of intact skin to any contaminated body fluids
- exposure via any route to body fluids other than blood, e.g. urine, vomit, saliva and faeces
- exposure to body fluids/blood from a source known to be negative for blood-borne viruses (HepB, HepC and HIV)
- for HepB virus exposure, regardless of the HepB status of the source, the member of staff/student is not at risk if they have shown an adequate antibody response following vaccination.

High risk exposures

- exposure to body fluids involving percutaneous injury, contact with broken skin or the mucous membranes
- exposure to blood/body fluids from a subject known or strongly suspected to be at high risk of being infected with a range of blood-borne viruses.
  Immediate action will be necessary based on the results of the risk assessment. Look for the appropriate protocol which should be widely available pinned to ward and GP surgery walls.

49) A Firm—a firm approach from the healthcare professional is more likely to gain a positive result
The principle behind brief interventions is that repeated, short, non-judgemental discussion surrounding an addiction will, with time, increase the probability of a patient making the decision to change. A paternal attitude is unlikely to achieve this.

FRAMES

- **F**eedback – assessment and evaluation of the problem
- **R**esponsibility – emphasis that the harmful behaviour is by choice
- **A**dvice – explicit advice on changing the harmful behaviour
- **M**enu – offering alternative goals and strategies
- **E**mpathy – the role of the counsellor is important

- **S**elf-efficacy – instilling optimism that the chosen goals can be achieved.

An alternative model for brief interventions is the 5As model:
- Ask – direct and/or indirect screening
- Assess – point on continuum, readiness for change
- Advise – educational feedback, CDC guidelines
- Assist – measures geared for preparation and action steps
- Arrange – follow-up, re-screen, referral

50) C SCOFF questionnaire

SCOFF is a screening questionnaire for eating disorders and is set out below:
1. Do you make yourself **S**ick because you feel uncomfortably full?
2. Do you worry you have lost **C**ontrol over how much you eat?
3. Have you recently lost more than **O**ne stone in a 3-month period?
4. Do you believe yourself to be **F**at when others say you are too thin?
5. Would you say that **F**ood dominates your life?

All the other questionnaires screening for alcohol problems:
- CAGE questionnaire – Cut down, Annoyed, Guilty, Eye-opener
- MAST questionnaire – Michigan Alcoholism Screening Test
- AUDIT questionnaire – Alcohol Use Disorders Identification Test
- SADQ – Severity of Alcohol Dependence Questionnaire

51) B Pregnancy

In any woman of child-bearing age with a period of amenorrhoea and abdominal symptoms, consider pregnancy. Acutely consider ectopic pregnancy.

52) A Alcoholic liver disease

First presentations of alcoholic liver disease may be subtle initially and can present in a variety of ways. Presenting features may include hepatic encephalopathy, jaundice, ascites (including spontaneous bacterial peritonitis), withdrawal, fits, haematemesis or bruising.

53) C Irritable bowel syndrome

Although irritable bowel syndrome (IBS) is a diagnosis of exclusion, NICE guidelines now include Rome III criteria as an aid to diagnosis.

Rome III criteria

A diagnosis of IBS should be considered only if the person has abdominal pain or discomfort that is either relieved by defecation or associated with altered bowel frequency or stool form. This should be accompanied by at least two of the following four symptoms:
- altered stool passage (straining, urgency, incomplete evacuation)
- abdominal bloating (more common in women than men), distension, tension or hardness

- symptoms made worse by eating
- passage of mucus.

Other features such as lethargy, nausea, backache and bladder symptoms are common in people with IBS, and may be used to support the diagnosis.

Management consists of explanation, fibre supplements, antispasmodics and antidepressants.

Red flag symptoms not typical of IBS

- pain that often awakens/interferes with sleep
- diarrhoea that often awakens/interferes with sleep
- blood in stool (visible or occult)
- weight loss
- Fever
- abnormal physical examination.

Irritable bowel syndrome (IBS) is a chronic, relapsing and often lifelong disorder.

54) C Painful macroscopic haematuria in an adult

Most men with lower urinary tract symptoms can be managed in primary care. Indications for urgent referral include:

- an elevated age-specific PSA in men with a 10-year life expectancy without signs of an active UTI
- microscopic haematuria in men over 50 years with irritative voiding symptoms
- hard, irregular, prostate swelling
- any evidence of acute renal failure or acute urinary obstruction
- normal but rising age-specific PSA with or without lower urinary tract symptoms (LUTS)
- persistent dysuria resistant to antibiotic treatment
- palpable renal masses.

55) E Otosclerosis

Otosclerosis often presents as conductive hearing loss in pregnancy and may be associated with normal tympanic membranes. It is due to fixation of the stapes footplate to the oval window and can be associated with blue sclerae. It can be treated with surgery and implant.

56) F Presbyacusis

Presbyacusis is also known as old age sensorineural hearing loss. Hearing aids are fitted when hearing is diminished in the low frequency range, i.e. range for TV, radio, phone and conversation.

57) B Herpes zoster oticus

When assessing hearing loss, look for evidence of vesicles in the canal as early aciclovir may shorten the attack and reduce long-term complications.

58) C Ménière's disease

Attacks are characterized by vertigo, hearing loss and tinnitus, nausea, vomiting and a feeling of pressure in one ear. Attacks can be treated with cyclizine and prochlorperazine. Recurrent attacks can be reduced using thiazides, betahistine and reducing salt intake.

59) A Acoustic neuroma

Acoustic neuroma is a slow growing schwannoma of the acoustic nerve. Consider this diagnosis in unilateral deafness and tinnitus. Facial palsy may also feature. An MRI of the internal acoustic meati should be carried out to diagnose or exclude acoustic neuroma. Treatment is with surgery.

60) C 25–49

Cervical screening is 3-yearly between ages 25 and 49 and 5-yearly between ages 50 and 64. In England, women between 25 and 64 years are screened. In Northern Ireland and Wales, women between 20 and 64 are screened. In Scotland, women between 20 and 60 are screened.

Note: The routine screening does not preclude smear testing in other age groups. This 21-year-old woman can certainly have a smear test done. She would not be automatically called for screening however.

61) E 50–70

The age range for breast screening is now 50–70 for the whole of the UK. The age range has increased from a maximum of 64 to 70, bringing England in line with the rest of the UK. The appropriateness of mammographic screening and an appropriate age range remains controversial.

62) B 12–13

At the time of publication the planned national immunization programme is to be for girls aged 12–13. From Autumn 2009, a 2-year catch-up programme will offer vaccination to all girls up to 18. All women should continue to attend for cervical screening. The HPV vaccines do not protect against all strains of HPV and it will be some time before a population benefit in cervical cancer rates will be seen. The vaccine is most effective if given before sexual activity starts.

63) E Sikhism

People of any faith or culture will vary in how they carry out customs. It is important to discuss relevant issues with individual patients.

64) A Practice based on personal experience

These steps were first described in 1992 as a model for carrying out evidence-based practice. They emphasize the need to discourage practice based merely on previous personal experience, and to look for robust scientific evidence.

The Sicily statement on evidence-based practice

1. Translation of uncertainty to an answerable question.
2. Systemic retrieval of best evidence available.
3. Critical appraisal of evidence for validity, clinical relevance and applicability.
4. Application of results in practice.
5. Evaluation of performance.

65) B 0.5 mL 1 in 1000 adrenaline

IM adrenaline (epinephrine) injections for anaphylaxis are of 1 in 1000 strength (1 mg/ml):

- less than 6 months, give 50 mcg (0.05 mL)
- 6 months to 6 years, give 150 mcg (0.15 mL)
- 6–12 years, give 300 mcg (0.25 mL)
- above 12 years, give 500 mcg (0.5 mL).

Each dose can be repeated every 5 minutes as necessary.

Adrenaline should be given immediately when anaphylaxis is suspected, while an ambulance is called. Indicators of anaphylaxis are laryngeal oedema, bronchospasm and hypotension. Chlorphenamine should be given orally or parenterally for 24–48 hours to prevent relapse. Hydrocortisone can then be given, though its onset of action is longer.

66) C 3 units

In the UK, alcohol units are measured as alcohol by volume. Units=% ABV × vol (litres), so
250 mL × 12% = 0.25 × 12 = 3 units.

67) A 1 unit

Units = % ABV × vol (litres), so 50 mL × 20% = 0.05 × 20 = 1 unit.

68) D 4 units

Units = % ABV × vol (litres), so 500 mL × 8% = 0.5 × 8 = 4 units.

69) H 20 units

Units = % ABV × vol (litres), so 500 mL × 40% = 0.5 × 40 = 20 units.

70) I 30 units

Proof is a measure of alcoholic content calculated as parts of alcohol in 200 parts of beverage. Therefore, an 80 proof beverage equates to 40% ABV. Proof is often referred to as 'percentage proof'. This is an inaccuracy as it is not a percentage. Units = % ABV × vol (litres), so 750 mL × 40% = 30 units.

71) A 1 unit
Where specific volume and ABV value are not given, estimate units via the traditional method of remembering a single shot of spirits is equal to 1 unit. The weakness in this system is that not all drinks have the same ABV.

Traditional alcohol unit guide

- pint of cider – 4 units (assumes 568 mL glass of 7% AVB cider)
- small sherry = 1 unit (assumes 50 mL glass of 20% ABV sherry)
- pint of beer = 2 units (assumes 568 mL glass of 3.5–4% ABV beer)
- glass of wine = 1 unit (assumes 125 mL glass of 9% ABV wine)
- measure of spirit = 1 unit (assumes 25 mL measure of 40% ABV spirit)
- bottle of vodka = 32 units (assumes 750 mL bottle of 43% ABV spirit)
- one bottle of wine = 7 units (assumes 750 mL bottle of 9% ABV wine).

Wine servings

- small glass wine = 125 mL
- standard glass wine = 175 mL
- large glass wine = 250 mL
- bottle = 750 mL

Beer servings

- bottle = 330 mL
- can = 440 mL
- pint = 568 mL
- litre = 1000 mL

Other servings

- spirits = 25 and 35 mL
- sherry = 50 mL 20%

72) D Continue normal daily activities and prescribe paracetamol
For simple mechanical back pain, aim to relieve pain and prevent disability. Opiates are rarely needed. Aim to discontinue after 14 days. Aim to stay at work as far as possible. Discourage bedrest. Assess for risk of depression, which can affect outcome.

73) B Arrange urgent referral
This patient has a series of red flag signs. Urgent investigation and referral should be carried out.

74) F Specialist referral if no better in 6 weeks after conservative management
This patient has nerve root pain, which should resolve with conservative management. If simple analgesia is inadequate, consider amitriptyline to treat nerve pain.

75) E Emergency referral
This patient has signs of a cauda equina syndrome (gait disturbance, saddle anaesthesia and sphincter disturbance) requiring urgent decompression. It occurs due to compression of the cauda equina below L2 level. He should be referred for emergency MRI. If this is caused by metastatic carcinoma, it must be treated by emergency radiotherapy. If a large prolapsed lumbar disc is the cause, it is treated with emergency surgical decompression.

76) C Assess for yellow flags
Yellow flags are associated with poor outcomes. Referral for reactivation/rehabilitation should be considered in patients who fail to return to work by 6 weeks.
Psychosocial 'yellow flags' in back pain include:
- a belief that the back pain is harmful or potentially severely disabling
- fear-avoidance behaviour and reduced activity levels
- a tendency to low mood and withdrawal from social interaction
- an expectation that being passive rather than active will help
- social or financial difficulties.

77) A An asymmetrical funnel plot suggests there may be publication bias
A funnel plot is a scatter plot used in meta-analysis. It plots study results against the size of the study. Where no bias exists, the plot should form a symmetrical cone about the mean result.

78) C Cervical carcinoma
The relevant risk age corresponds to the target age for cervical smear screening.

79) A Uterine carcinoma
Carcinoma of the body of the uterus is less frequent than cancer of the cervix or ovary. It must be excluded in any case of postmenopausal bleeding.

80) D Vulval carcinoma
Can present very late due to non-presentation in the affected age group. May present as a fistula or may arise from postmenopausal lichen sclerosus.

81) A Endomysial antibodies

In a child with such developmental failure and gastrointestinal symptoms, coeliac disease must be excluded. None of the other tests would be either very sensitive or specific. Endomysial antibodies are around 90% sensitive and 100% specific. In this setting, exclusion of gastrointestinal infection via stool samples is prudent. Treatment of coeliac disease is lifelong withdrawal of all gluten-containing products. These include wheat, barley and rye products. Coeliacs have a varying tolerance to oats. In any case, it is important that the oats do not contain traces of other cereals, for example from contamination from within the same factory.

82) A Autosomal dominant

83) A Autosomal dominant

84) C X−linked recessive

85) E Polygenic inheritance

86) B Autosomal recessive

87) A Autosomal dominant

88) E Polygenic inheritance

89) C X−linked recessive

90) B Autosomal recessive

91) D X−linked dominant

92) E Polygenic inherituned

It is a good idea to memorize the mode of inheritance of the most common genetic disorders. If you do not know the answer to a question, there are some rules of thumb to bear in mind:

1. If you have not ever considered the condition to be genetic, it is likely to have polygenic inheritance.
2. Next, consider if you have ever heard of a condition being sex-linked. If so, it is likely to be X-linked recessive. There are very few well known X-linked dominant conditions other than Rett syndrome and vitamin D resistant rickets. X-linked recessive conditions will be expressed in males and females but with a greater incidence in females due to the greater number of X chromosomes.
3. This then leaves autosomal conditions. If the condition causes mainly structural signs and symptoms, it is likely to have autosomal

dominant inheritance. If the condition causes mainly endocrine or metabolic problems, it is likely to have autosomal recessive inheritance.

4. If you have never heard of a condition, it is likely to be rare and so is most likely to have autosomal recessive inheritance if it is a single gene defect.

Try these rules out on the list above.

It is also time well spent revising the features of the most common genetic conditions, e.g. those whose features are listed in the *Oxford Handbook of General Practice*.

93) C Lung carcinoma

94) B Colorectal carcinoma

95) A Breast carcinoma

Cancer mortality, 2005

- lung   22%
- colorectal   10%
- breast   8%
- prostate   7%
- others   53%

96) E
Cancer mortality in males, 2005

- lung   24%
- prostate   13%
- colorectal   11%
- oesophagus   6%
- others   46%

97) A
Cancer mortality in females, 2005

- lung   19%
- breast   17%
- colorectal   10%
- ovary   6%
- others   48%

98) D Unplanned pregnancy
Age, ethnicity and education do not affect risk of domestic abuse. Although income level does not generally affect risk, living in poverty or poor living conditions increases risk. It is important to remember, however, that anyone can be at risk of domestic abuse, male or female.

Risk rises in pregnancy and if already a sufferer, abuse tends to increase in pregnancy.

Risk factors for domestic abuse

- when attempting to leave an abusing relationship
- poverty
- unemployment
- disability
- social isolation
- previous abuse as a child or in a relationship
- witnessing abuse as a child
- pregnancy, especially if unplanned.

99) B History of alcoholism
Risk factors for becoming violent in a relationship
- current abuse of alcohol or drugs
- was a victim of, or witnessed abuse as a child
- history of abuse of previous partners
- unemployed
- abuses pets.

100) C 1–year history of cardiac failure with atrial fibrillation
The gynaecomastia is likely to be due to having been prescribed digoxin for his cardiac symptoms. Other drugs causing gynaecomastia are spironolactone, cimetidine and metronidazole. Daily headaches suggest potential prolactinoma. Unexplained lethargy could be attributed to renal or liver failure, both of which can cause gynaecomastia. Tumours producing androgens (or HCG, or oestrogen) cause gynaecomastia.

Gynaecomastia is a growth of the breast tissue. Apparent gynaecomastia in obese people can be confirmed as breast rather than fat tissue only by clinical examination.

References and further revision resources

Back IN. *Palliative Medicine Handbook*, On-line Edition. Penarth: Pontypridd and Rhondda NHS Trust, 2008. http://book.pallcare.info.

Bandolier. *Knowledge Library*. Oxford: Bandolier, 2008. www.jr2.ox.ac.uk/bandolier.

Bentley P. *Memorizing Medicine: A Revision Guide*. London: RSM Press, 2007.

Boland W. Alcohol and primary care. *InnovAiT*, 2008; 1: 2.

Cancer Research UK. *CancerStats*. London: Cancer Research UK, 2008. http://info.cancerresearchuk.org/cancerstats.

Department of Health. *The Ionising Radiation (Medical Exposure) Regulations 2000*. London: DoH, 2007. www.dh.gov.uk.

Department of Health. *New GMS contract*. London: DoH, 2007. www.dh.gov.uk.

Department of Health. *Know your units*. London: DoH, 2008. www.units.nhs.uk.

Department of Health. *The gold standards framework: A programme for community palliative care*. London: DoH, 2008. www.goldstandards framework.nhs.uk.

Department of Health. *The UK immunisation schedule*. London: DoH, 2008. www.immunisation.nhs.uk.

DVLA. *At a glance guide to the current medical standards of fitness to drive*. Swansea: DVLA, 2008. www.dvla.gov.uk.

Egger M, Smith GD, Schneider M, Minder C. Bias in meta-analysis detected by a simple, graphical test. *BMJ* 1997; 315: 629–34.

GPnotebook. Cambridge: The Cambridge Institute for Medical Research, 2008. www.gpnotebook.co.uk.

Health and Safety Executive. *Reporting of Injuries, Diseases and Dangerous Occurrences Regulations*. London: Health and Safety Executive, 1995. www.hse.gov.uk/riddor/guidance.htm.

Health Protection Agency. *Infectious diseases, chemicals and poisons, and radiation*. London: HPA, 2000. www.hpa.org.uk.

Jones R, Latinovic R, Charlton J, Gulliford MC. Alarm symptoms in early diagnosis of cancer in primary care: cohort study using General Practice Research Database. *BMJ* 2007; 334: 1040.

Lewis S, Clarke M. Forest plots: trying to see the wood and the trees. *BMJ* 2001; 322: 1479–80.

National Institute for Health and Clinical Excellence. *NICE guidances*. London: NICE, 2008. www.nice.org.uk.

NHS Cancer Screening Programmes. *Cancer Screening Programmes*. Sheffield: NHS Cancer Screening Programmes, 2008. www.cancerscreening.nhs.uk.

NHS Scotland. *NHS Scotland and Confidentiality and Data Protection Website*. Edinburgh: NHS Scotland, 2008. www.confidentiality.scot.nhs.uk.

Nicholson TRJ, Cutter W, Hotopf M. Assessing mental capacity: the Mental Capacity Act. *BMJ* 2008; 336: 322–5.

Pendleton D, Schofield T, Tate P, Havelock P. *The Consultation: An Approach to Learning and Teaching*. Oxford: OUP, 1984.

Riley B, Haynes J, Field S. *The Condensed Curriculum Guide: For GP training and the new MRCGP*. London: RCGP, 2007.

Royal College of General Practitioners. *Good Medical Practice for General Practitioners*. London: RCGP, 2002. www.rcgp.org.uk.

Royal Pharmaceutical Society of Great Britain. *British National Formulary*. London: BMJ Group and RPS Publishing, 2008. www.bnf.org.

Scottish Intercollegiate Guidelines Network. SIGN guidances. Edinburgh: SIGN, 2008. www.sign.ac.uk.

Simon C, Everitt H, Kendrick T. *Oxford Handbook of General Practice*, 2nd edn. Oxford: OUP, 2006.

UK Border Agency. *Asylum and refugee status*. London: Home Office, 2008. www.ukba.homeoffice.gov.uk.

Young C. (ed.) *BMJ Clinical Evidence Handbook*. London: BMJ Publishing Group, 2008.

Keyword index